CROSSCORE®
HARDCORE

REVOLUTIONARY RESISTANCE:

HOW TO BUILD MAXIMUM MUSCLE AND EXTREME STRENGTH WITHOUT WEIGHTS, MACHINES OR GYMS

MARTY GALLAGHER

AND

Chris Hardy D.O. CSCS WITH Michael Krivka

CROSSCORE® HARDCORE

REVOLUTIONARY RESISTANCE:

ISBN 10: 1-942812-05-1   ISBN 13: 978-1-942812-05-0
This edition first published in June, 2016
Printed in China

Book design by Derek Brigham • www.dbrigham.com • bigd@dbrigham.com
Photography by Tai Randall

— TABLE OF CONTENTS —

For those of us that are honored to call Marty Gallagher our friend, we know him to be a no B.S. guy that just happens to have been a national and world champion in both powerlifting and Olympic weightlifting. He was also a national and world championship team coach. He is a trainer and mentor to many of the world's most elite athletes. He is also a trainer for elite Tier 1 Spec Ops military types, both here and abroad.

Gallagher has an ability to forge the human body from what it is into something far better, through the expert use of iron and steel. It is quite something to watch him work his magic and it would be impossible to find a resume as impressive and proven as his. Whether you're a newbie wanting to transition your physique from flaccid to hard, or a seasoned athlete that wishes to improve upon their already awesome level of fitness and athleticism, Gallagher is the man to see.

Marty was asked by some of his elite spec ops buddies a few years back, "Is there a portable training device out there worth a damn!? Can a real Man get a real workout using a portable training device?" This was the query that was the genesis for this book. During his search for a deep deployment fitness tool he came across the CrossCore®. The versatility and uniqueness of the tool caught his attention and he "took it to the woodshed." He emerged with a strategy he dubbed, CrossCore® HardCore.

He expropriated Old School barbell and dumbbell "modes and methods, techniques and tactics" and applied them to the CrossCore®.

He then "test flew" his Old School strategy with this newest of tools by distributing units and instruction to his network of elite strength athletes, spec ops fighters, secret agent government types. He wanted to make sure real men could in fact get real workouts from this lightweight portable training tool. The Gold Standard for resistance training workouts is barbells and dumbbells. The CrossCore® needed to replicate the results derived from Gold Standard tools.

The feedback was superlative—we knew we were onto something.

One particular chapter in this book hit a particularly resonant chord with me, "Ghosting" Operator X Thru A CrossCore® HardCore Workout." Marty uses his storytelling abilities to present a great example of what we witnessed time and time again: top athletes actually using the CrossCore® in the way it was intended. Their facial expressions morph from pure skepticism into dawning acceptance before ending in wonderment. Even those with the highest level of training and conditioning can be brought to their knees when this tool is melded with Gallagher's tactics.

As co-inventor of the CrossCore® and having a longtime passion for weightlifting, it was truly exciting for me the day Marty contacted us and wanted to vet the CrossCore® for his Spec Ops guys. I knew who Gallagher was, and it's not everyday a writer and thinker of his caliber relates, after giving the tool a shakedown cruise, that he is dead serious about creating a new protocol to complement our new tool.

It was as if we had invented the Marshall amplifier and stack and the Fender Stratocaster guitar—and here came Hendrix.

Marty Gallagher is to CrossCore® Rotational Bodyweight Training what Jimi Hendrix was to the electric guitar. For those of us that know Marty, I'm sure we're all smiling at that comparison. Both are great examples of the awesomeness that can be created when the right mind connects with the right tool at the right time.

Genius extracts things and ideas from these tools that we mere mortals never imagined.

J.P. Brice – Ironcompany, Forged Passion™ Since 1997

CROSSCORE® HARDCORE

INTRODUCTION

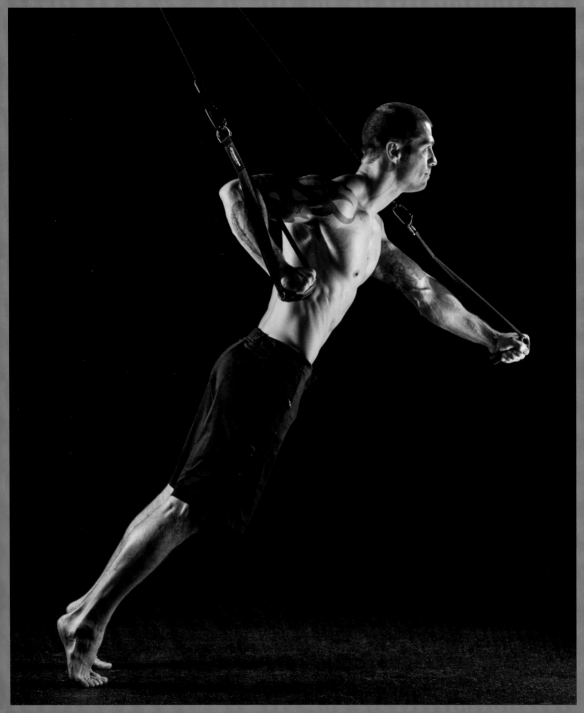

THE FITNESS HERETICS

n the movie, *The Wild One*, Marlon Brando's character was asked, "Johnny, what is it you're rebelling from?" His sardonic retort, "What do you got?"

We are fitness heretics. We too are rebelling. We willfully puncture holes in mainstream fitness shibboleths. We challenge assumptions that have become so sacred that no one is allowed to question the "settled science" upon which these mythological fitness commandments are founded.

Over time, the sacrosanct commandments of mainstream fitness have become brittle, fossilized, predictable and static—yet apologists conveniently overlook the inconvenient truth that the exercise protocols and recommended diets of the mainstream champions never came close to delivering the promised results.

Livelihoods and entire industries have been built upon these sacred fitness doctrines, yet despite negligible results these ineffectual methods have become institutionalized and entrenched. Lockstep orthodoxy in exercise and diet has created fitness industries, fitness conglomerates and a veritable religion, a fitness religion based on belief, faith and unquestioning conformity rather than science, empiricism and actual results.

We are the fitness heretics. What are we rebelling against? What do you got?

We will diverge from the mainstream strength training orthodoxy on virtually every topic, idea or philosophy. Our path is guided by cold science and real results: our system is rooted in the cumulative collective empirical experience of our world champion and world record holding strength mentors: we were mentored by hall of fame strength athletes and we in turn have mentored world champions and hall of fame strength athletes. That our system works is beyond dispute.

Our methodology is not static or fossilized. Our only allegiance is to tangible physical results. Let us be clear: our goal is simple and profound: the radical transformation of the human body.

Ultimately, the reason people undertake a fitness regimen is to renovate and transform the human body: they seek to melt off excess body fat, build and strengthen muscle, improve health, increase endurance and amp up their vitality.

Our philosophical path has a mind of its own and we follow it wherever it takes us.

We consciously, conscientiously and continually gather new information, data gleaned from the elite athletes we train on a regular and ongoing basis. We examine and analyze new data obtained from the training trenches; we weave pertinent new ideas, strategies, tactics and tweaks into the organic, ongoing strength and fitness narrative.

Our strategies are rooted in cause and effect, science and empiricism. Our report card grade is based on our ability to elicit tangible, measurable, quantifiable results on a consistent and continual basis.

Our system is all about attaining strength, power and muscle. A considerably stronger athlete is a considerably better athlete. Our resistance training approach has been in existence, in differing evolutions, for 70 years. The philosophic tenants were formed in the 1940s and improved upon by each succeeding strength generation. Atop a venerable Old School strategic foundation, we have layered additional strength wisdom accumulated and acquired in the interceding half-century, leading up to the present.

Elite athletes swear sole allegiance to the flag of tangible progress. Mainstream fitness "experts" and defenders of the fitness status quo, question the importance of obtaining actual results. Mainstream fitness experts form a clique that downplays its inability to generate real results for regular people by suggesting that results are overrated.

In pretend fitness, everyone gets a participation trophy; in elite athletics, results are all that matters.

FORCED PHYSICAL EVOLUTION: STRUGGLE AND EFFORT
THE FUNDAMENTAL TRUTH OF EFFECTIVE RESISTANCE TRAINING

The elite are privy to the insider knowledge: superhuman effort is needed to create the spark that ignites the transformative fire. Herculean effort, nothing less, is needed to attain resistance critical mass and force the body to change and adapt—think about it; adding muscle is a *defensive* act that only occurs in response to extreme bodily trauma and perceived threat.

The body creates new muscle fiber or enlarges and strengthens existing muscle fiber, only in response to the body-shocking, self-inflicted trauma caused by hardcore, progressive resistance training. The body will only morph itself in response to extreme training; the body adds muscle as a way of adding more protective 'armor' for defense against future attacks.

Here is an amazing fitness factoid and one routinely (conveniently?) overlooked by mainstream fitness experts: without intense physical effort there will be no results; in order to create muscle and power there need be tremendous effort—otherwise there is no reason, no incentive, nothing of any significance, to *force* the body to react to an event (training) so extreme that the human body is *compelled* to reconfigure itself.

This is profound. Wrap your head around this fundamental resistance training fact: pure physical effort is the nucleus, the spark, the irreducible central event needed to elicit the results we seek from our *resistance* training efforts—we need resistance, and lots of it, in order to force the evolutionary changes we seek.

John Q. and Mary J. Public never come remotely close to generating the degree of sheer physical effort (intensity) needed to set the spark that initiates "the process." Physical transformation is not an event—it is a process. The degree of pure hellacious effort required is beyond the comprehension, capacities and capabilities of normal fitness participants.

The well-meaning, fitness-minded normal folk that "exercise" at the local Y, health spa or commercial fitness facility, generate modest physical effort resulting in modest physical gains. Typically, mild efforts have a nice initial effect on an untrained body. However once the wondrous initial four to six weeks' timeframe is complete, the untrained body is no longer untrained: from this point forward to trigger true physiological gains the degree of effort must be increased exponentially.

Civilian fitness trainers mistakenly surmise the same exercises done in the same way and in the same fashion, exerting the exact same level of intensity will continue to generate astounding results indefinitely. In reality, past the first six weeks and any physiological gains to be realized from a beginner training regimen has long since been realized.

Unfortunately, the misinformed civilian takes away the wrong message. Rather than correctly surmise, "Hey, this little initial burst of physical progress is over—let's retire this stale training routine and rotate in a fresh and vibrant strength and muscle-building protocol; one that will shock my body out of this complacent status quo. Let's make a conscious effort to increase the degree of difficulty." Struggle, effort and intensity are not to be avoided, rather, sought out and embraced; there is an irrefutable relationship between struggle and transformative gains.

At some point, the current level of effort and intensity is no longer sufficient to generate the gains sought. We need to find new ways in which to shock the body out of its current complacent state. Instead of embracing the logical conclusion that something new and different is needed, fitness trainees become fitness zealots: "I *know* this resistance regimen works because it worked for me!"

Indeed, it worked wonderfully for six weeks, but then again, practically any training system, no matter how lame or inane will work wonders on an untrained body—for a short while. When someone that has not lifted weights or performed any cardio suddenly begins to exercise religiously four to five times a week, that person will harden up and shape up. Add in any crazy diet and you have a recipe for some nice initial progress—but the name of the game is *continual* progress and initial progress is easy.

Continual progress springs from innovation, not fossilization.

There are those that—having experienced a sweet, short, burst of fantastic initial progress—now swear Hitlerian allegiance to whatever training template they happened to be using initially. They now treat the "system" as if the tenets were the sacrosanct commandments from a fundamentalist religion. Any deviation is heresy; the system is deified and always done the same way in the same fashion and done without question. It is comfortable and enjoyable to perform the same exercises for the same number of reps using the same poundage in the same way, ad infinitum, for weeks, months and years, never changing a thing.

Those that refuse to change, can, at best, hope their modest, sensible training maintains whatever initial gains they made in those glorious first few weeks. Doing the same thing over and over and expecting different results is a form of insanity, yet dogmatic thinking is rampant and dominant in mainstream fitness. The mainstream contends that meek and mild training can elicit fantastic results. Plus, meek and mild is far safer and less strenuous and straining. If fitness is eviscerated of its vital essence of effort, transformation devolves into ritual or game.

OLD WINE IN NEW BOTTLES;
OLD METHODS USED WITH NEW TOOLS
CAN BRUTAL AND SIMPLISTIC WAYS
BE APPLIED AND ADAPTED TO HI-TECH TOOLS?

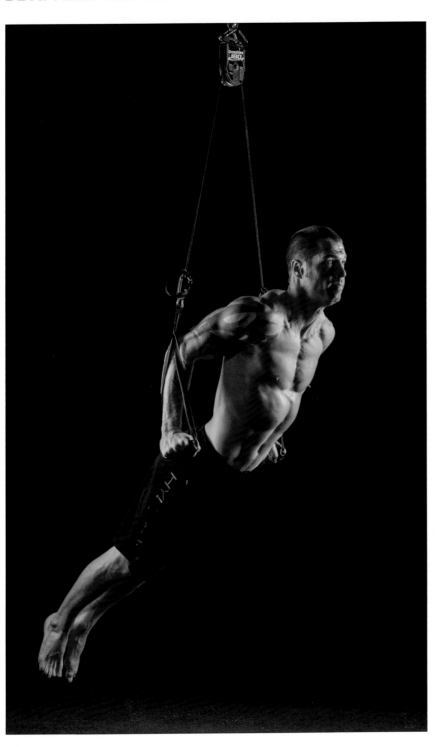

The goal of this book is to relate a highly effective method for eliciting dramatic resistance training results—using an exciting portable training device: the CrossCore®.

We have created a strength-training/muscle-building strategy for the CrossCore® based on our extensive hardcore barbell/dumbbell background. We have developed a series of extremely specific exercise techniques to be used in conjunction with a series of highly defined training protocols.

The end result is giving purpose to a wild new training tool, unlike anything anywhere in fitness. We provide the techniques and tactics that enable the intelligent trainer to turn the m into a devastatingly effective tool, a tool that weighs less than five pounds and fits inside a bag the size of a loaf of bread.

After prolonged and extensive testing on ourselves, we then tested out our embryonic strength strategies on our world champion athletes and our active duty elite military commando buddies. The results were and continue to be, outstanding. So much so that we created this book to share with the wider world the sensational results the elite were attaining using these modes and methods.

A few years back we were asked by our military friends to vet portable training devices. Our elite clientele wanted to know if any portable training device could be used in such a way as to deliver results comparable to the type and kind of results derived from gold standard barbell/dumbbell free-weight progressive resistance exercises.

This book is the explanation of how and the affirmative answer to that query.

PART I

ORIGINS AND FOUNDATIONS

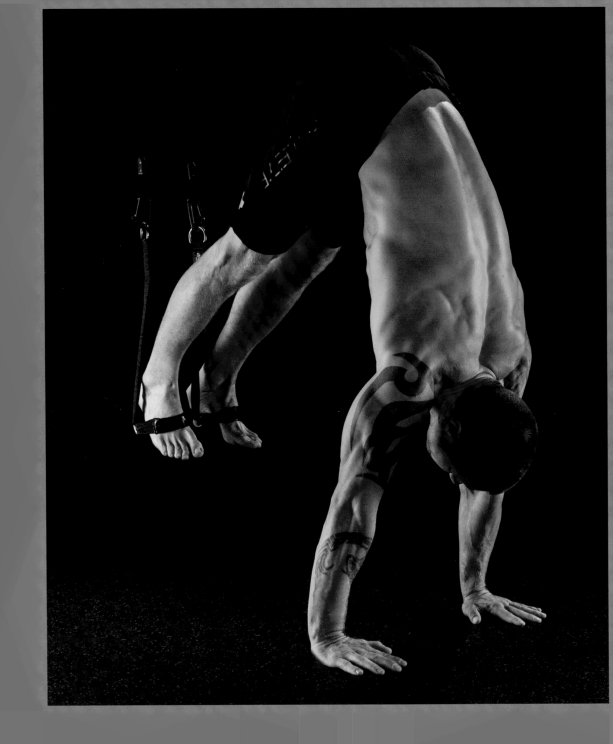

GOALS, TOOLS, PROTOCOLS AND MOTIVATION

WHO WE ARE, AND WHY THAT MATTERS

"Effective resistance training triggers tangible physiological results: we successfully strengthen targeted muscles, we improve measurable performance in any and every athletic benchmark, we transform the human body as we forcibly morph ourselves; we become significantly stronger and significantly more muscular. To achieve success, combine perfect techniques with hardcore training tactics. Train like your hair is on fire; train with incredible intensity and consistency. Intensity and consistency are mental traits."

—Hugh Cassidy, World's first powerlifting world champion

That paragraph contains a lifetime of collective training wisdom. Cassidy's dictum has guided our hardcore resistance efforts since 1968, so it seemed only logical and natural that we attempt to apply his fundamental precepts to this new fitness tool.

Could we create an effective resistance training protocol that retained the transformative essence of Cassidy's transformative prescription? We would need to narrow down the mind-boggling potentialities of the CrossCore®—as the device (in full rotational mode) presented so many exercise possibilities that it was potentially either paralyzing or diffusing.

Cassidy's resistance training strategy makes mention of the mental aspects of hardcore resistance training—and empirical experience has shown that the hardest single attribute to acquire in any transformational fitness regimen is *motivation*. With motivation there is hope for transformation; without motivation there can be no transformation. There is no such thing as a casual dramatic physical transformation. To radically change our physiques requires radical action.

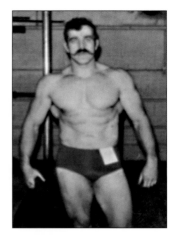

Those that ultimately succeed in building a better body are those that positively burn for transformation. Motivation grows out of an intense dissatisfaction with how a person looks and feels. From intense dissatisfaction grows intense motivation. People who are thoroughly dissatisfied (disgusted?) are those that likely will generate the sustained motivation needed to power the process.

Being dissatisfied and motivated is not enough: without a tool and plan a goal becomes a wistful dream. The lucky dissatisfied find the golden needle in the fitness haystack and stumble onto a tool and a protocol that will actually enable them to favorably reconfigure their physique—while simultaneously improving capabilities, capacities and performance.

The CrossCore® is a highly versatile device that is being used to dramatically improve cardiovascular capacity and increase strength/endurance. The CrossCore® can be used to extend and enhance mobility, flexibility and pliability; the CrossCore® shows incredible promise as a rehabilitation tool for medical professionals. There are endless uses for CrossCore® and these meaty topics deserve in-depth discussion at another time.

Our particular area of athletic expertise lies in making humans significantly stronger: increased strength invariably produces new muscle tissue and dramatic increases in strength prefigure equally dramatic increases in human performance, regardless the benchmark selected.

The purpose of this book is to share an extremely effective Old School hardcore muscle-building strength-infusing protocol that has been modified for use with the CrossCore®. We have dubbed this adaptation of the Cassidy strength theory, CrossCore® HardCore.

The CrossCore® HardCore methodology is a descendant of a venerable strength method handed down to us by world champion strength athletes—our athletic mentors. In turn, we have mentored world champion strength athletes, using these same ancient protocols. These primal strength strategies have now been amplified with our own hard-earned empirical knowledge—the wisdom that comes from winning national and world titles and coaching national teams to world team titles.

When it comes to effective, result-producing resistance training, we know of what we speak. This tool—used properly—can trigger hypertrophy, improve raw strength and power and open up an entire new universe of untapped rotational strength potentialities. We have the protocols if you have the motivation.

CROSSCORE®
MILITARY ROOTS

"CAN A REAL MAN GET A REAL WORKOUT USING A PORTABLE DEVICE?

"We are what we do repeatedly"

—Aristotle

Every Sunday afternoon, I field phone calls from around the country and around the world. In addition to elite military, I also work with Jack Bauer-types that operate within governmental counter terrorism units. One commonality all the warrior types have is they all have to travel quite a bit, and are often stuck for protracted periods in locales without training facilities. One longtime spec ops friend used to regularly call me from Afghanistan late Sunday afternoon. It would be nighttime and his squad would be gathering together to head out on yet another snatch-and-grab mission.

For four months of every year this Tier 1 pro, a man with twelve straight combat tours, was dispatched to some godforsaken hellhole to chase bad guys while alternately freezing or frying in inhospitable climates. He related that while deployed he experienced unending bouts of boredom interspersed with nightly missions often ending in violence and fury. It was a life of extremes.

The missions were repetitive: take a helicopter ride to the middle of nowhere in the middle of the night, arrive at a jump off spot, sneak up on the bad guys humping 70-pound packs for eight to ten kilometer hikes that usually ended with a mountainous ascent in order to successfully creep up on a village. The squad would then leap out, grab and handcuff the Taliban dude(s) then hike back out to the jump off point to be picked up by the helicopter, captives in tow. There was always apprehension and tension and sometimes gunfire and killing.

He'd call in the boring minutes before the night mission kicked off and we'd talk about resistance training. He had suffered a horrific back injury during a mountain climbing training exercise accident. We had designed a resistance program that "trained around" his injured back yet was a serious, uncompromising strength training regimen. His back may have been jacked—but as he would tell me when I tried to baby him, "There is nothing wrong with my arms, legs and most of my back." We found ways to tax, strengthen and power-ize his undamaged body parts.

One Sunday afternoon he called and was bitching about the lack of fitness equipment of any kind at the locale he was stuck in for the next four months. He asked if there were any portable training devices that could be used as a serious resistance tool. Were there any portable training tools able "to give a real man a real workout?" By 'real workout' he meant a workout that could replicate the strength, power and muscle growth results attained using barbells/dumbbells and power training.

Was there a portable training device that could realistically replicate results obtained from gold standard resistance tools? I told him I didn't rightly know if such a tool existed, but I sort of doubted it and would do my best to find out. His initial inquiry led to my eventual discovery of the CrossCore®.

I was the ideal person to vet a portable resistance-training device as I was a super skeptic and my hunch was that portable training devices would prove insufficient and inconsequential. I would be fine reporting back just that: "Sorry men, they all suck and they all are worthless—at least insofar as resistance training applications." I would have had zero compunction relating that, if it turned out to be the case.

Could the CrossCore® be used by a serious trainee as a high-yield resistance-training tool? Could we recreate the requisite degree of muscular stresses needed to trigger the miracle of cellular reconfiguration? Proper resistance training creates significant and sustained hypertrophy for a protracted period: would the desired results be transferable? Could I ascribe and assign to the CrossCore® the spectacular results we were realizing from our hardcore barbell and dumbbell training? I would not compromise on results: the CrossCore® would have to trigger the body's adaptive response—and as a man with 50 years of hardcore resistance training under my belt, I would know results when I saw them.

Maximally intense exercise is, unfortunately, the only exercise that causes the human body to favorably reconfigure itself; only super human effort is enough to force the body to grow muscle; this type of resistance training has a devastating physiological impact on the body.

The mistake the orthodox fitness types make is they try and find ways to avoid or lessen this devastating impact. The core truth of physical transformation is this: the physical devastation, the trauma, is responsible for the adaptation, the miracle of muscle growth and all the newly acquired power and strength. Take away the intensity and effort and there is no trauma; without that pure physical devastation you eviscerate the effort and ruin the results.

When using the CrossCore®, would it be possible to create the requisite resistance, the degree of difficulty, the sufficiently intense muscular effort to trip the hypertrophy switch? I would make that determination on an exercise-by-exercise basis.

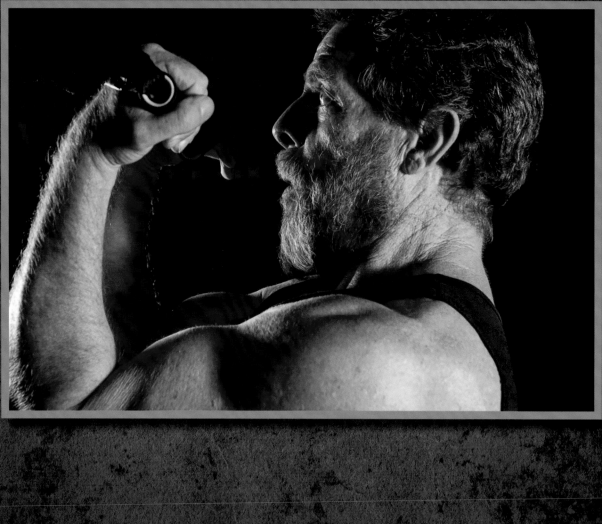

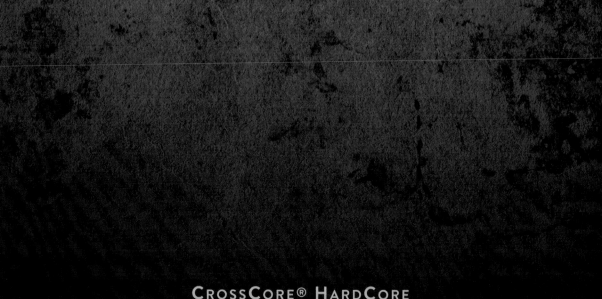

CROSSCORE® HARDCORE

TIME TO TRAIN:

WHERE THE RUBBER MEETS THE ROAD...

*My CrossCore® journey begins with arm work and is
highlighted by the unexpected appearance of endorphin nirvana-bliss*

I attached my first ever CrossCore® to the chin bar and grabbed the handles. Now it was time to actually put this device through its paces. All the thoughts had been thought—I was seeking something very narrow and specific from the CrossCore®. I would test this tool with cold empiricism. I didn't care about the CrossCore's® aerobic capacities, or the CrossCore's® value as a flexibility enhancer or as a rehab tool, I didn't care about the cool gymnastic moves you could perform. I only cared about one thing: could I create and replicate a series of resistance training exercises and could I generate the requisite payloads that would duplicate results obtained from free-weights?

For four months of every year this Tier 1 pro, a man with twelve straight combat tours, was dispatched to some godforsaken hellhole to chase bad guys while alternately freezing or frying in inhospitable climates. He related that while deployed he experienced unending bouts of boredom interspersed with nightly missions often ending in violence and fury. It was a life of extremes.

On what particular exercises? Done in what way? How often? How long? Sets and reps? So many legitimate questions that needed to be answered if I were to create a protocol that would enable the CrossCore® to morph into a kick-ass resistance training tool. In my very first home gym training session using the CrossCore®, I performed two exercises: bicep curls and triceps extensions. There is something quite natural about performing curls using the CrossCore®, particularly in pulled-pin mode.

As you stand and look at the device, a handle in each hand, it seems the most natural thing in the world to lay back, plank the torso and with palms facing upward, curl the rigid body towards the handles and anchor-point using both arms or one arm at a time. It took me a few sets of curls to figure out my optimal curl technique. I also played with foot placement: I wanted to fail in less than ten reps while using a grind rep speed and a full range-of-motion.

I found out that I could make CrossCore® curls maximally taxing with great ease. I could increase the CrossCore® curl "payload" by inching my heels forward ever so slightly; I could lighten the CrossCore® curl payload by inching my heels backwards ever so slightly; thereby lessening the angle, and ergo, lessening the payload.

After a few minutes of working alone in the solitude of my garage, I found a perfect heel position, one that enabled me to perform five perfect single-arm curl reps utilizing pristine technique. When I curled using this device I was able to lock in on a bicep isolation movement pattern that was maximally taxing and maximally isolating. I could, quite literally, make my biceps contract over every inch of the concentric and eccentric rep stroke.

As I pulled each of these strange, single-arm steep layback curls to completion, my biceps felt as if they were going to burst through the skin. I found that on curls, the CrossCore® could give me all the resistance I could handle. Once I became comfortable with the strange, suspended-in-space curl technique, I found I could maneuver my body in such a way that I could tax and attack the biceps from angles I had never before thought of, much less experienced.

I could alter the payload up or down, heavier or lighter, during the actual rep. Imagine, you are struggling with the fourth of five reps. You know there is no way you will successfully complete the fifth rep. Using barbells or dumbbells that set would be over. With the CrossCore® you have this unique ability to inch your feet back a few inches, thereby instantaneously lightening the curl "payload." No need to stop the set, simply inch forward or backward and keep repping! I felt this was a huge plus for the CrossCore®.

Would not repping past the point you would ordinarily have to quit be a good thing? Physiologically speaking? From a hypertrophy-inducing standpoint, would it not be better to continue the set, consciously and instantly reducing the poundage, allowing the athlete to continue to rep and take the set deeper and deeper into the hypertrophy zone? This approach actually has a long lineage in progressive resistance training and is expressed as "drop set" strategies. The drop-set approach would figure large in my emerging template.

My overarching idea was to expropriate Old School training tactics from hardcore resistance training and use these strategies with the CrossCore®. I would mimic heavy dumbbell work, taken from hardcore power training and apply these strategies to the CrossCore®. I came to love one particular CrossCore® curl protocol. Using this CrossCore® curl protocol, I found I could dig a muscular inroad as deep and thorough as any I had ever experienced using gold-standard dumbbells.

My CrossCore® curl strategy called for me to wear out each bicep individually—then continue curling with both arms, until I could not complete another rep. I sought utter and complete bicep failure. This technique was actually an adaptation of the "drop set" principle that has been used by iron masters as a resistance-training tactic since the 1950s.

A proper dumbbell drop set would have the lifter rep out, perhaps curling a pair of dumbbells, using pristine technique. The lifter would curl with a particular poundage until they could curl no more; when they had achieved "positive failure," the curler would rack the dumbbells, immediately grab another pair of bells (a good 30% lighter) and without pause rep the lighter bells to failure. Done, he would rack this set of bells and immediately commence a third and final drop set with an even lighter pair of bells. Rep out, drop the poundage rep to failure yet again, drop the poundage (yet again) and rep to failure one final time.

If a man were capable of curling a pair of 50-pound dumbbells for five strict reps in the standing dumbbell curl, he would do just that, curl a pair of 50s until he got four (bad day) or five (good day) perfect curl reps. He barely makes the fifth rep and sets the 50s back into the dumbbell rack. He immediately grabs a pair of 35-pound dumbbells and curls them to failure. Let us assume he makes five clean reps with the 35s. He now racks the 35s and immediately begins a third and final drop set, repping out with a pair of 30s or 25s.

For the CrossCore® drop set, rep out in the two-armed, pulled-pin, bicep curl. Ideally we seek to find a foot placement and body angle that causes us to reach failure in five reps. Let's assume you complete five perfect two-arm curl reps. Without pause shuffle your feet backwards three to six inches. This decreases the curl payload and you continue repping, ideally you complete five more curl reps with the reduced payload. Shuffle backwards one final time, making the CrossCore® curl poundage lighter yet. Perform a third and final set of five + curls.

You have just completed a CrossCore® three-phase drop set. This drop-set protocol is referred to as the "foot-shuffle drop set."

I found another way in which to replicate a drop-set protocol by using a combination of single arm and double arm curls combined with a grind rep speed, relaxation, and a full range of motion. The strategy was to "rep out" on each arm, then finish off curling with both arms to failure: we start with the weak arm and perform a set of five curls. Optimally we "dial in" the resistance as the one-arm curl set unfolds and the fifth rep (ideally) is so taxing and demanding that rep six is an absolute physical impossibility.

You can't do another curl with your weak arm so you now switch to the strong arm and ideally you hit positive curl failure on rep five with the strong arm. Now begin curling with both arms, curl with great deliberation and curl with both arms until you cannot perform another two-armed curl.

The "drop" in drop set is expressed by suddenly shifting from curling the entire bodyweight of the torso with a single arm, to curling the entire bodyweight of the torso with both arms. This tactic keeps the set going. I noted how when I began curling with both arms, though the weight was lighter the burn was so intense that I had to stop on the 6th rep using both arms. My arms were fried: I was shaking, flushed and maximally pumped. I was shocked at how difficult this curl sequence had been.

I immediately flipped over without pause and began performing triceps extensions. I was doing a classical 'free weight" bicep/triceps super set and used the same procedure on the triceps extensions that I had used with the curls. My triceps extensions were done one arm at a time before finishing the set with two arms.

I leaned forward, facing away from the anchor-point. I unlocked my left arm and lowered down. The upper arm stays stable and next to the ear; only the forearms move to lower and extend. Done right, the tricep targeting in the CrossCore® is superb; you can play with slight body and arm positioning adjustments that enable you to isolate the triceps to an amazing degree: providing enough payload to stress the triceps was also no problem.

I "repped-out" with my weaker left arm, hitting positive failure on a barely completed, grind-speed fifth rep. I then repped-out using my stronger right arm, again going to positive failure, again using the grind and again barely making it to rep five. On my second rep on my right arm tricep extension, I sensed the payload was too light. I intuitively felt I could likely do eight to ten reps with my stronger right arm. So I slithered backwards, perhaps six inches. Placing my feet closer to the CrossCore® anchor-point even a few inches made the payload considerably heavier. I was able to get six reps with my right.

I continued the set by repping with *both arms*, I repped until another rep was impossible. I made seven excruciating, triceps-burning, two-armed tricep extensions before hitting the wall. My triceps, like my biceps, were engorged and inflated, blood-filled, swollen and red, both biceps and triceps bursting through the skin.

I knew this feeling; this was the same feeling I would get after an absolute maximum set of heavy dumbbell curls, drop-set style, alternated with drop-set triceps pushdowns. Both biceps and triceps had been maximally taxed in a single, perfect, extended CrossCore® extended set. The degree of muscular exhaustion was profound and astounding.

This "One-and-done" strategy worked so well and was so effective that there was no need for any further training of the targeted arm muscles. When successfully subjected to this particular protocol, the targeted muscles are so blasted, so taxed and so exhausted, that further working of those muscles is not only ineffective and superfluous it is downright counterproductive.

Like the CrossCore® curls, the CrossCore® tricep extensions were extremely intense: each rep started from a deep and relaxed triceps pre-stretch position. From this maximally stretched and relaxed position, the rep transitioned into maximally contracted "hard lockout" at the conclusion of each and every rep. On both curls and extensions, the horrific "grind" rep speed was used. Slowing a rep down amplifies the degree of difficulty, to a dramatic degree. After one set of biceps and one set of triceps, my arms were devastated, brutalized, burnt to a crisp as surely as if I'd used a pair of dumbbells. I now knew I could replicate free weight techniques using the CrossCore® and I could create payloads sufficient to tax the strongest of men: this was a fantastic discovery. The CrossCore® was a resistance revelation.

ACCESSING THE ADRENALINE/ ENDORPHIN AXIS OF EXCELLENCE

After having just blasted my arms to total exhaustion in less than 10 minutes performing a lone, extended set of biceps and a lone extended set of triceps, I now gazed with satisfaction at my swollen arms. As I caught my breath, a familiar afterglow descended and took ahold of me; I floated off into an exercise-induced endorphin nirvana. I was in a familiar bliss zone. I stayed there most of the rest of the afternoon. The appearance of endorphins signified the degree and depth of inroad, the intensity generated during the actual CrossCore® exercise.

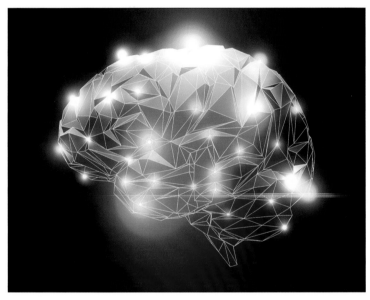

The appearance of endorphins was evidence that the degree of effort exerted was sufficiently intense to trip the high-threshold hypertrophy switch. I was *thrilled* to be able to cause endorphins to secrete using the CrossCore®. I now knew that, at least when training arms, I could create resistance sufficient to trigger endorphin release. The appearance of endorphins after my CrossCore® arm training session was a positive indicator and a profound testament to the effectiveness of the effort. Elite athletes have long known about the unique relationship between intense exercise and endorphins. Intense effort releases endorphins and accelerates the production of testosterone and growth hormone. Science, per usual, is behind the curve.

1. On the front end of the session, *adrenaline* lifts workout performance. Elevated workout performance creates and releases endorphins into the bloodstream

2. The degree of endorphin release is in direct proportion to the severity of the effort; the harder and more prolonged the training effort, the greater the endorphin secretion

3. The appearance of endorphins signifies that the degree of effort was sufficient to trigger muscle growth, hypertrophy. Concurrently comes additional power and raw strength

4. Muscle growth requires intense physical effort. The shattered muscle is fed and rested and not trained again until recovered: train, eat, rest—this constitutes the "growth cycle"

Metabolic 'Amping' occurs as a direct result of an intense progressive resistance training session. Truly intense training has an acceleratory affect on the metabolism. An amped-up metabolism is highly beneficial; whereas an obese couch potato has a sluggish metabolism, the champion athlete has a metabolism that rages like a tramp freighter's boiler under full steam. The athlete's metabolic thermostat stays elevated for hours after ending a hardcore training session. Calories are burnt at an accelerated rate; body fat is mobilized and oxidized, as fat is used for fuel after glycogen is exhausted.

Now the question became: how many other CrossCore® exercises could I identify where we could create the same superb degree of intensity and difficulty as we created with the biceps and triceps? What other CrossCore® resistance exercises could be made difficult to the degree that they induced hypertrophy and in doing so unleashed telltale endorphins?

Could we effectively train quads and traps with the CrossCore®? How about delts or hard-to-hit hamstrings? Which muscles could the CrossCore® maximally tax and which ones would the device be unable to stimulate? There was zero doubt in my mind that exercise effectiveness, using the CrossCore®, would vary, radically and dramatically, exercise to exercise, body part to body part. You might be able to decimate arms, but how are you going to isolate and blast the erectors?

My quest was to create clones of those super-effective Old School resistance exercise techniques I knew so well. How many classics could be replicated using the CrossCore®? If I could replicate the techniques, could I provide sufficient payload? The goal was to be able to use the CrossCore® to increase power, strength and muscle—to replicates gains obtained from a free-weight workout. If I could create a catalog of CrossCore® exercises that reasonably duplicated classical free-weight exercises, my deployed friends could get a kick-ass, no-compromise, resistance-training workout from a portable training device. Now that would be a hell of a good thing.

I identified and then attempted to mimic a broad range of free-weight exercises using the CrossCore®. I created cloned techniques and applied as many hardcore barbell/dumbbell training tactics and strategies as were feasible. My idea was to create a CrossCore® resistance protocol that would replicate, as near as possible, the barbell/dumbbell strength systems used successfully by elite iron athletes for eons. I sought to create movement patterns and protocols that mimicked barbell and dumbbell techniques and tactics. I coupled these technical replication movements with "amplified" payloads and melded techniques with Old School periodization power tactics—we would use old methods with a new and different tool.

Over time, I developed a "hardcore protocol" for the CrossCore®. I mimicked hardcore progressive resistance exercise techniques on the CrossCore® while simultaneously creating payloads significant enough to tax elite athletes. In doing so, we would obtain the results nominally obtained from expert use of hardcore free-weight barbell and dumbbell exercises using the CrossCore®. That was the goal.

A year later, I was training a group of thirty active duty spec ops warriors, including my friend that had originally asked about portable training devices. We were putting on a five-day extended seminar/workshop and part of the presentation was a section where Dr. Mike Davis and I demonstrated the CrossCore®. We were presenting the CrossCore® as an effective resistance-training tool for use when deployed. Mike Davis, DPT is one of the nation's leading physical therapists and our dual presentation was called, "Portables for deployment—worth the effort?"

I wanted to share with these military elites the protocols I had devised for this new resistance-training device: the CrossCore®. We wanted to use a volunteer and demo our resistance training protocol for this strange new tool in front of the larger group. What better way to communicate how to perform a workout than to witness a successful and suitably intense workout?

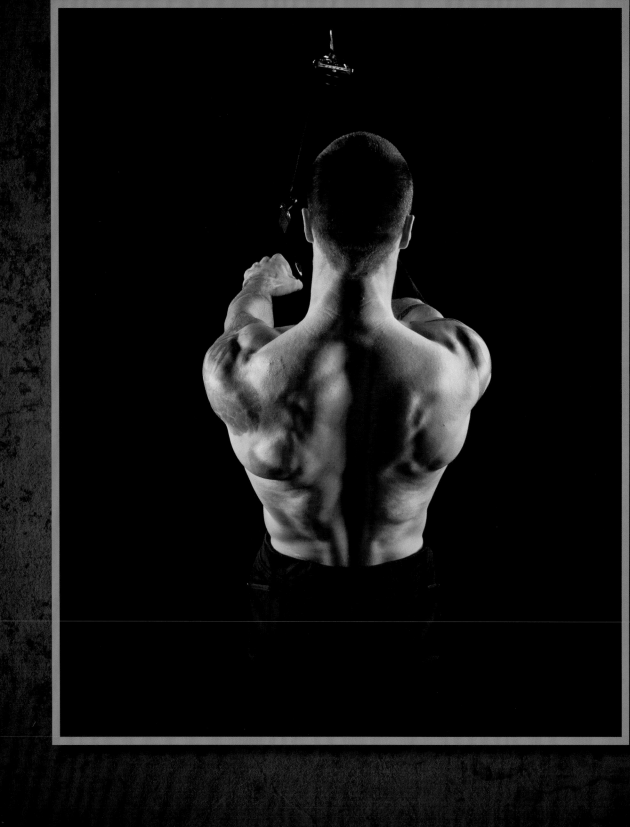

"GHOSTING" OPERATOR X THRU A CROSSCORE® HARDCORE WORKOUT

"THIS ISN'T WHAT I'D EXPECTED... THIS IS A HELL-OF-A-LOT BETTER THAN I EXPECTED!"

The CrossCore® weighs four pounds, fits in a small black bag and can be backpacked anywhere. We found that we could replicate a vast number of classical free-weight exercises and further, we could create payloads for those free-weight-mimicking, full range-of-motion movements that could bring the strongest of athletes to positive failure in 10-reps or less. We took several CrossCores® with us on this five-day military seminar. "Doc Mike" (as the soldiers call him) and I were intent on putting a super soldier through a CrossCore® hardcore resistance-training workout.

Mike is a tough critic; very thoughtful, analytical and a tad cynical—which is a good thing. When we compared notes we found that we had arrived at similar conclusions: our initial consensus was that the CrossCore® was no joke. Both of us were particularly excited by the CrossCore® when it was used in full rotational mode; we had each developed specific modes and methods for our own purposes. We had both gotten the results we sought for ourselves: now it was time to see if we could provide these same results to others.

We wanted to have skilled athletes to test drive the CrossCore® using my embryonic HardCore resistance training protocols. Since Mike and I just happened to be in a large gym stuffed full of elite athletes, we recruited one of the best, a man with ten straight combat tours under his belt. A super-soldier. He would test drive the CrossCore® using our HardCore protocol to determine if this resistance training tool was worthy of lugging on deployment.

Operator X is an active duty sniper and extremely fit. He stands 5-10 and weighs a thick 205. Before each CrossCore® exercise we instructed our Spec Ops fighter on exactly what we expected him to do. We had specific techniques. We sought to stymie a dude that was in the top 1% of the top 1%. Operator X was skeptical. He wryly noted that most fitness devices were one-dimensional toys, hardly worthy of lugging to some remote hellhole. On deep and extended deployments, most spec ops operators intent on a workout are resigned to free hand exercise, using bodyweight for resistance. The CrossCore® fits inside a 10-inch bag and weighs less than five pounds. If it could do the job, it was the right size and weight.

In this particular session, Mike and I decided to target pectorals; latissimus dorsi, front, side and rear deltoids; rhomboids and teres; biceps and triceps. The strategy would be to utilize perfect techniques in conjunction with payloads significant enough to force this strong man to involuntarily curtail the set, regardless the exercise, somewhere in the magical five to ten rep range, the ideal rep range for inducing hypertrophy and increasing strength. As muscle maestro Bill Pearl once said, "A muscle does not care what *mode* or *tool* is used to induce hypertrophy—just as long as hypertrophy is induced, what matter how?"

Operator X was hard, lean and compact. He was built like a football free safety while most of his compatriots were somewhat taller and not near as thick and powerful. X grinned as he examined the CrossCore®, "So you really think this f@#king toy can give me a real workout?" He was obviously skeptical.

Doc Mike is a friendly stoic, a man of few words. He motioned to X to grab the handles. I described the contents of the first "extended set" we wanted X to perform. This first round would consist of five exercises, strung together, back-to-back and done non-stop. This was to be a low rep, size and power affair, Old School resistance training designed to pack power and muscle onto his pecs, shoulder, mid and upper back, biceps and triceps. And we were going to get through the entire workout in 15 minutes.

X was dubious when we told him we were going to physically burn him down. He laughed. "Not f#%king likely..." In the interest of time, efficiency and as a test of our "non-conflicting" exercise sequence strategies, Operator X would perform a protocol consisting of five exercises, a giant set, one set of each exercise, done in rapid-fire succession...

1. Chest press pectorals (upper and lower) front delts, triceps
2. Row upper and lower lats, teres, rhomboids, rear delts
3. I-Y-T raises front, side and real delts, traps, rhomboids, teres
4. Bicep curl inner and outer biceps
5. Tricep extensions three tricep heads

Operator X was a strong boy with a 350-pound paused bench press. If we were to bring him to positive failure, we were really going to have to "disadvantage'" his leverages. The trick would be to provide him sufficient resistance. In order to make every rep maximally difficult and maximally effective, we insisted operator X...

1. Use "Grind" rep speed: push and pull purposefully slow, powerful, non-explosive
2. Use one limb then the other limb then both limbs (excepting I-Y-T)
3. Use full and complete range-of-motion on all exercises without exception
4. Use ultra-specific exercise techniques: precise pathways repeated consistently
5. Use pauses: a dead-stop at the rep "turnaround" amplifies the degree of difficulty
6. Use full and complete lockout on every rep of every set

The first exercise was the chest press and this was the CrossCore® exercise I worried most about being able to tax X. He was benching 350 and had copious amounts of raw rugged power. It was time to begin.

I wanted to give him as radical an angle as possible. I sought to make his payload as heavy as possible. "Set your feet here." I indicated a foot position close to the fulcrum. With a big, strong man, we start with steep angles that force them to lift the largest possible percentage of their bodyweight on every rep.

If allowed to push explosively with both arms, X likely could do 30 + reps, even using the most extreme angle. We needed to slow down his roll. The first "intensity amplifier" we would use would be to implement a slowed, "grind" rep speed. The second way in which to make the exercises more difficult was to have him use a single arm at a time. Finally, we added a relaxed pause at the bottom of each bench rep—it all heaped more difficulty atop the already tough one-arm chest press.

We began with five reps—strict, slow, precise reps using the weaker arm, paused and sunk at the bottom of each chest press rep. Then he did five chest press reps using his strong arm, sink and pause. He finished with as many reps, grind speed, paused and sunk, he could get using both arms. X got seven clean two-arm chest press reps before being unable to push another rep. Every excruciating rep was done with great concentration, evenness and deliberation.

When he unlocked his elbow to begin his first chest press rep. I verbally told him what to do; I wanted him to replicate our single-arm dumbbell power bench press technique. I verbally guided him. "Don't *lower* yourself down using gravity, *pull* yourself downward using power and precision. Keep the elbow *in* as you lower. We want the handle to end up next to the bottom of the pecs at the low point." X pulled himself to the low position of the chest press; his right arm stayed locked and straight as he lowered his torso until his left fist was next to his armpit. His body was nearly parallel to the floor. He had lowered down as far as possible.

During the lowering, per the classical free-weight, strategy, he inhaled. He was full of air, chest fully expanded at the bottommost point. I gave him his next instruction. "I want you to exhale, relax the muscles of the chest and arms and sink into the handle." He did so. This little technical twist created a pause and the purposeful relaxation caused a "pre-stretch" condition.

To shift from relaxing and stretching a muscle into a maximal contraction creates optimal muscle fiber stimulation. It all combines to make any exercise far more difficult—which is what we seek. We are looking for ways to cause a 350-pound strict bench presser to fail in less than ten reps without using a barbell.

X was at the bottom of his first rep in the chest press, one arm straight and flexed while his left arm was totally relaxed. He sunk into the handle without losing position. "Feel the stretch! This is like iron yoga." It was time to press. "Don't jolt or jerk when you shift from stretch/relax to pushing erect: use a slow and smooth application of pure power." He began to push upward. He was "grinding" to lockout. His rep speed was slowed, but just a tad, nothing ridiculously slowed, I call it 'barely slow,' yes we slow down the rep speed, but we don't overdo the slowing or it destroys payload handling ability.

He pushed his body upward one grind-inch at a time. "Make sure and lock the elbow hard at the conclusion of the bench rep." As he straightened his left arm, I emphasized. "Harder lockout! Really straighten the arm and lock the elbow." What I didn't mention was that this little trick of the resistance trade caused maximal flexion and contraction of pecs, front delts and triceps. He went on to complete five of these magnificent grind reps with his weak arm. I noted that his left arm was shaking as he locked out rep five. That is a good sign of intensity and degree of effort. I wouldn't say he couldn't have gotten another rep or two with this arm, but we weren't done just yet.

I instructed him to repeat the chest press process, now using the strong right arm. He began repping and on rep three I actually had him shuffle backwards a few inches as the "weight" seemed light and I wanted to increase the payload. He was pressing too easily. This minute adjustment made his strong arm pushing instantly more difficult. He was exhibiting the telltale signs of shaking in his right arm as he locked out the fifth rep with his right arm.

I instructed him to, without pause, commence chest pressing with both arms. Now he commenced two-arm pause-and-stretch chest pressing, lowering and raising himself with the same deliberateness he exhibited using one arm. Because he now pushed with both arms, he effectively slashed his payload in half—however he was pushing on fried arms. Now he understood why we started with the weaker arm; it was allowed to recuperate during the time the strong arm pressed.

We had reduced his chest press payload dramatically, yet by the time he was commencing his fifth rep, his tattooed arms shook as he lowered, they shook while he relaxed paused and sunk, and they shook like palm trees in a hurricane as he barely locked out rep five. "You are done pressing. Let's row."

A properly performed dumbbell row is a topflight back exercise. I wanted the CrossCore® row technique to be the mirror image of the CrossCore® chest press technique. This was a "push/pull" philosophy expropriated from hardcore barbell/dumbbell training: work either side of the human torso—pecs and lats—and optimally we work each side of the limb with an *identical* technique: the chest press was a push while the lat row is a pull. Optimally, both are done identically. I sought Operator X to row using as close to the same motor-pathway he'd used chest pressing.

I spoke to him as he turned and faced the CrossCore® anchor and reset his hands in the handle. "I want you to think of these rows as 'reverse chest presses.' We want to use the identical technique you used on the chest press for the row: same arm position, same rep stroke pathway, same rep speed; same everything only instead of pushing a load, you'll be pulling the load." Using the identical protocol used on chest pressing,

Operator X began by performing five strict rows using his weaker left arm. He was instructed to lower with control and tension, at the bottom, relax, release the tension thereby enabling the body to sink and the lats to stretch even further. Now, maximally relaxed, I had him commence a slow, controlled, methodical pull until the left handle hit his left pec. That was one rep, by the fifth rep, using this precision technique, he was gritting his teeth.

He switched hands and began rowing with his stronger arm. I had him shuffle his feet forward roughly four inches: I calculated this would make the strong-arm row payload a good 10% heavier. When he barely completed the fifth rep with his strong arm, Mike instructed him to commence rowing using both arms.

The tendency is to speed up the rep speed or bounce at the turnaround, when the rep gets tough. The human body and brain seek ways to slip past, avert, avoid, side-step or make easier sticking points. Our strategy was to *create* sticking points using the CrossCore® and then power through these sticking points with technical integrity. Or fail with integrity. That was alright too: what was not alright was to purposefully seek and find and implement cute little slick ways to make sticking points not so sticky...conquering not-so-sticky sticking points might give the illusion of improvement—but resistance training infected and riddled with ease is an eviscerated training art.

At the top of each row rep I had X pull his elbow *behind* his torso. The slow grind and full range-of-motion made these five row reps tough pulling. I slipped around behind him and noted that his working lat was undergoing various flexions as he rowed; his biceps were staying relaxed and he was making an excellent mind/lat connection.

Five one-arm row reps with his left arm, then five reps with the right arm. He was stronger on the right side, so I had him shuffle towards the pulley to make the rows a tad heavier. Done rowing with his strong arm, he now began five grind row reps using both arms. As he ended the second two-arm row rep, X inched himself forward without prompting: he was self-accessing that the payload was too light. He finished his row set, weak arm for five reps, strong arm for five reps, then both arms. On the final two-armed row phase X caught fire and rather than stop at five reps, went on to perform eight hard fought reps before being unable to perform and ninth two-armed row.

We had been able to create the requisite techniques and the requisite degree of difficulty for Operator X in both the chest press and row. No small feat as this was a strong dude. We needed to keep the resistance party going. Having blasted chest and lats, it was a perfect time to attack the deltoids, plus the smaller muscles surrounding the shoulder blades, including the traps. I had devised a three-phase deltoid exercise that was superbly suited to the CrossCore®. I dubbed it the "I-Y-T."

This is a three-phase deltoid raise: three distinctly different versions of the same exercise. X set his feet and layback to begin the "I" portion of I-Y-T. He would perform five reps in each phase.

The "I" was accomplished by raising his arms directly overhead. From a plank layback facing the CrossCore® anchor, X would allow his arms to go limp. The fists were palm down, straight ahead, the two hands were within six inches of one another; they would stay this close together throughout the front raise phase. From this relaxed start position, the fists would be raised together directly overhead. The "I" portion of the exercise replicated a heavy *front raise* in classical progressive resistance training. Done right, a proper front raise builds and strengthens the front delts; it also stimulates teres, rhomboids and causes a surprising degree of trap flexion.

As Operator X began to rep the "I" phase, I reminded him to "Replace explosiveness with deliberateness." As he began repping, it looked way too easy so I had him increase his payload by moving his feet forward a full six inches at the beginning of the second rep. All of a sudden he was struggling—perfect! He maintained his form and barely completed his fifth rep. Done with the heavy front raise, it was time for the Y phase.

The Y phase illuminated an unforeseen benefit of the CrossCore®: as Doc Mike called it, "the ability to work 'in between' two classical exercises." In conventional weight training, the shoulders, the deltoid region, can be expertly exercised using a pair of dumbbells—front raises, lifting two bells, one bell or a tightly held barbell plate from crotch height to overhead while keeping the arms straight, has a profoundly stimulating effect on the front deltoids, a sliver of triangular muscle wedged next to the pec.

The rear and side deltoids, the outer delt heads and the monster rear delts, are equally stimulated by a proper set of side lateral raises or bent-over rear lateral raises. There exists a motor-pathway that is neither a side-lateral nor bent-over rear lateral...this pathway falls "in between" each movement and is accessible only through the use of the CrossCore®.

The "Y" movement, done on the CrossCore®, requires the athlete take his clenched fists, each holding a CrossCore® handle, from the crotch to overhead with the fists three feet apart at the top of the rep. The technical trick is to use a very specific motor pathway, a Y pattern. The fists holding the handles (palms down) start off low and together and are raised overhead, up and out, keeping the arms straight. This Y pathway hits both front and side delts to a degree unobtainable using free weights. The odd angle and disadvantaged leverage causes the strongest of men to struggle with low reps done at grind speed.

Again, when X barely completed the fifth Y rep, Mike and I smiled. This was tough work and the cumulative effect was starting to show—so far, in our extended and not completed set, we had done one and two armed chest presses, rows, Is and Ys, each set taken to a tough, hard-fought conclusion. Without moving his feet or pausing, Operator X began the "T" phase of this three-phase delt and upper back exercise. This exercise essentially mimicked a bent-over rear lateral raise, only done standing. The T phase required five reps and on each rep the fists were pulled rearward, parallel to the floor, handles slung wide at the end of each rep.

X was getting the hang of the device and shifted his feet a few times without being prompted. He was "dialing in" the payload. He knew that the goal was just a hair shy of positive failure—or as we call it, "positive-failure-minus-one." We encouraged him to shift around to make things harder or easier, whatever was called for, whatever was needed to make a set stall before 10 reps.

He used pure strength and muscle to complete his reps, no momentum, no rebound, no fudging through sticking points; it was easy to make it difficult for him to perform the I-Y-T on the CrossCore®: the leverage is poor and using low-speed torque maximally engages rear delts and mid-back. During the contraction phase, no matter how difficult it became, X didn't contort, speed up or break form in order to slip through the muscular sticking point. We sought out muscular sticking points and powered through them—that was where the hypertrophy was and that was where the strength gains resided. X struggled to complete his fifth rep in this slowed-down, reverse flye.

Done with I, Y and T, it was time to hit the arms. I noted his condition. He was a fit super athlete, so he wasn't going to display exhaustion or go to one knee or start bitching or gassing out. On the other hand, we wanted him to struggle in order to be able to barely complete the final reps in each phase of each exercise. So far in this one extended set he had no less than nine maximal efforts—in eight minutes.

Time for arms...having given 100% effort (or more) in each of our three multi-phased rapid-fire exercises, Operator X's chest, shoulders, upper back and lats were pumped and exhausted, it was as if he'd been lifting weights. While maintaining his rowing stance, Operator X extended his arms, leaned back and flipped his palms skyward. He now began to curl. He began curling with his weak arm using the gruesome grind speed. He dug in and made a foot adjustment. As he curled, he lifted his elbow higher, purposefully making the curl harder. He knew he was doing it right because he felt an intense contraction in his left bicep during every inch of every left arm curl rep.

He kept pulling on every curl until his clenched fist passed his ear. This was a "continuous tension" curl; he lowered with great deliberateness, feeling the negative, at the bottom of each curl relaxing and allowing his bicep to stretch. From this relaxed pre-stretch, he methodically curled his torso upward, creating a bicep contraction so intense he thought his bicep would burst though the skin. He made five perfect curl reps.

After five curls with the weak left arm, he began to curl using his strong arm. Per usual, he made his 'strong side' curls a bit heavier by shuffling forward ever so slightly. Operator X was becoming adept at modulating the payload in order to make the set end with a maximum effort on a final pre-determined rep. Done performing five tough reps with each arm, he now shifted, without pause, to two-arm curls.

By using both arms he made the payload lighter, effectively replicating the drop-set iron protocol. X was becoming an expert at increasing or decreasing the payload as the set progressed in order to purposefully 'gas out,' i.e. barely making that final predetermined rep.

Regardless the CrossCore® exercise selected, by altering the foot position or the technique we are able to "make the exercise heavier." This ability to increase or decrease the resistance "in flight" during a rep enables the smart and attuned trainee to provide just the right amount of resistance to cause the body to fail on the ideal appointed predetermined rep.

As we got deeper into the curl set, X instinctively put an arch in his back to isolate the biceps even more. I had him supinate his wrists at the top of each curl: as he curled he lifted his elbows *and* turned his wrists outward during the "loaded" portion of each curl rep. He barely made his fifth and final two-arm curl. He actually had to scoot backward during the fifth and final rep as he needed to lighten his curl load if he was to complete five reps without breaking form.

 He completed his final double-arm curl, stood erect and caught his breath. After fifteen seconds, he had normalized. He flipped around and now facing away from the CrossCore® anchor began to perform one-arm triceps extensions. As was the custom, he lowered his weaker left arm to begin the set. He performed five single-arm reps for each arm. He then concluded with six reps using both arms.

Mike and I insisted Operator X keep his elbows tight to his head throughout his triceps extensions. "Don't let the elbows flare outward!" I admonished. "Letting the elbows flare lessens the degree of difficulty the triceps are subjected to, a trick that allows us to slip through the sticking point—which is exactly what we do not want." X finished his triceps extensions and stood erect. He was flush-faced as he peeled the handles off his hands. He beamed. "That was f@#king *tough!*" Tough was the highest compliment. "I loved that sequence! That was an ass kicker all day long!"

He had completed the five-phase extended set: chest press, row, I-Y-T, curl, tricep extension in 12 minutes and 22 seconds.

The muscles we had trained were decimated. Our 33-year old spec ops fighter was pumped, swollen, flush-faced and breathing hard after going through our CrossCore® five-exercise Giant Set sequence. Operator X had been converted from cynic into believer. "I am liking this! This isn't what I expected—this is a hell-of-a-lot better than I expected!"

Operator X felt that the CrossCore® "used like we used it" made the grade and would find a place in his gear on his next deployment. After the short workout, X was exhausted and exhilarated; he was experiencing the post-workout endorphin rush, the hormonal nirvana that accompanies intense free-weight training and only occurs in response to a workout sufficiently intense. X offered up a ringing endorsement. "That was a seriously good chest/shoulder/arm workout! This tool used in this way blasted the hell out of me. I wouldn't have believed it if I hadn't experienced it."

Our work was done. We had created another convert to the CrossCore® Hardcore strategy. And we hadn't even touched on the pulley exercise dimension or the fact that the CrossCore® can be used to create intense strength/endurance workouts.

Yet another question loomed large: even though we were able to elicit results from elite soldiers and elite strength athletes, could we translate this embryonic CrossCore® HardCore methodology and make it effective, doable, user-friendly and applicable for a normal person living a normal life? We were amazed and pleased with how easily the untutored regular person was able to use our core tactics. The techniques are easily learned by anyone with access to a CrossCore®.

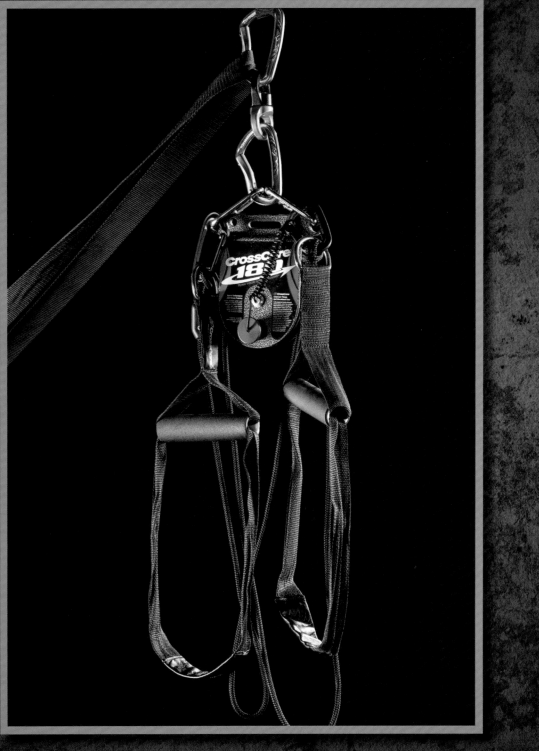

PART II

TECHNIQUES
AND TACTICS

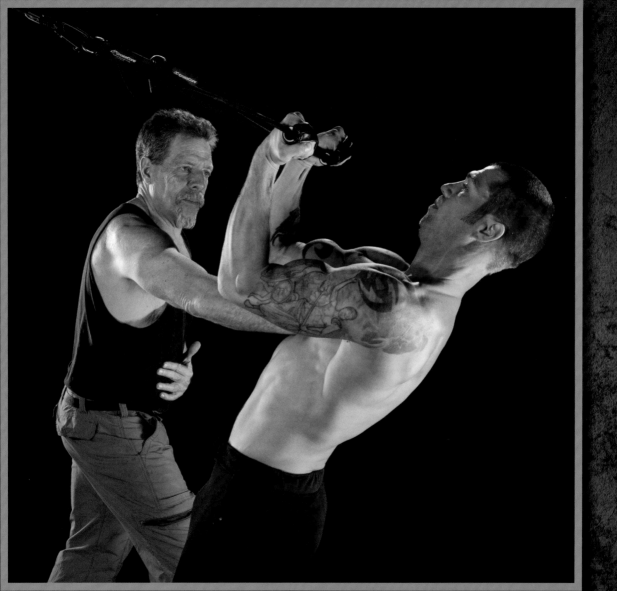

CROSSCORE® HARDCORE RULES AND PRINCIPLES

"SIMPLE IS AS SIMPLE DOES." THE GUMP-LIKE STRENGTH PHILOSOPHY OF "DOING FEWER THINGS BETTER."

We practice a "purposefully primitive" resistance training strategy that is primal and sparse. Ours is a sophisticated minimalism. We advocate, "doing fewer things better." We select a few critical resistance-training exercises and perform the selected ones with great care, precision and expertise. When we narrow the exercise menu, we are making a commitment to excellence: we raise exercise technique to an art form.

By confining ourselves to a select few exercises, we find ourselves doing these movements often, thereby allowing us ample training opportunity to hone and improve our technical skills; we focus on feel and develop proficiency in a few, select movements. We worship at the altar of technique. We know the technical archetypes and we seek to replicate these idealized techniques with ever-greater exactitude. Once we have built our sparse arsenal of extremely specific techniques, we turn our attention to tactics.

The specific techniques required of the CrossCore® Hardcore Protocol are non-negotiable if you want to see results:

1. Make the mind-body connection to push past the brain's fatigue protective mechanism and maximize intensity
2. Look to meet or exceed capacity on any given training day. This is a moving target
3. Training should be intensity-based, not volume based
4. Use "grind speed"
5. Utilize "intensity amplifiers"
6. Make use of the "third dimension of tension"
7. Achieve the "barely completed repetition in every set"

1. OVERCOMING THE BRAIN'S "CENTRAL GOVERNOR", TO MAXIMIZE INTENSITY

Once we have learned our archetypical techniques, once we have selected our exercises and decided on a tactical template, it is time to train. We now have our techniques and tactics and the question becomes—what degree of effort need be exerted in order to trip the hypertrophy switch?

How do we trigger the magical, mystical "adaptive response," how do we cause the condition wherein the human body transforms in response to training stimuli? How do we know when we have trained hard enough?

Champion athletes couple cutting-edge techniques with sophisticated tactics and great genetics to which they then add a ferocious mindset. Exposure to world-level athletes and Tier 1 Special Operations operators on a continual basis allows us to note certain commonalities. One obvious champion trait is mindset: when training, elite athletes and operators have an ability to exert at 100% of capacity (or more) on a continual and consistent basis.

Our brain is hardwired to protect us. It will shut down the body if a stimulus is perceived "dangerous." Noted sports medicine researcher Tim Noakes has described this phenomenon with endurance athletes. It applies to resistance training as well. The brain can override the body when threat is perceived. A body free of an overprotective brain can perform light years beyond what is thought possible.

This does not mean that we train through an injury or break technique—as that can be injurious. We can generate unbelievable intensity if we unshackle the body from the brain's protective mechanisms against fatigue. Special Operations soldiers do this all of the time during their training.

Topflight athletes understand that the way to improve overall athletic performance is to improve the quality of the individual workout. The goal is to string together an unbroken series of spectacular training sessions, each subsequent workout better than its predecessor. The athlete uses a series of successful sessions to create physical and physiological momentum leading up to the event or competition.

The best athletes *attack* their workouts; they train fierce, they are impassioned and engaged; during a training session the elite routinely "will" the body to exceed actual capabilities and capacities. They are able to override the protective "central governor" in the brain to increase intensity in the face of fatigue, while maintaining pristine technique. Focus and willpower are developed and used to elevate the intensity and quality of the workout. This ability to focus and concentrate in order to elevate workout performance is a skill that improves with time and practice.

A man with sophisticated techniques and state-of-the-art tactics—but with a lackadaisical, pre-occupied, unfocused mind—will fail. Conversely, using a lesser system—but powered by an extreme mindset—can lead to success...exuberant athletes usually prefer the outward berserker psyche while quieter personalities might psyche with an iceman mindset. The point is to seek some sort of physiological transformation. Training is not balancing your checkbook or a gentle diner party; the best training has some sort of heightened arousal aspect that creates far greater gains than those obtained by the lackadaisical sophisticate.

THE ADAPTIVE RESPONSE IS ONLY TRIGGERED IN RESPONSE TO SUPER-HUMAN EFFORT

Let us put a finer point on "super-human effort." If we work up to our capacity, regardless the exercise or technique, physiologically you have done all you can do. What more can a trainee do, other than work up to, or past our current limit?

Every time we complete a limit rep, every time we exert so much that we are unable to perform another rep, we have done all that we can do. Literally, you have repped until you are unable to perform another rep—that is equaling or exceeding capacity. What more can you do?

On a good day, you might succeed in exceeding your all-time best effort in a particular athletic expression or activity. On a bad day you might be off a full 20%. Yet even on an off day, you can still push or pull up to and past your limit. An elite trainee can always train to their limit, regardless if their limit on that particular day is enhanced or diminished.

From a hypertrophy and strength-building standpoint, better to hit 102% of diminished capacity on a bad day than 82% of enhanced capacity on a perfect day; even though that 82% might exceed 102% in terms of actual performance.

Back in the 1960s our world champion strength mentors taught us that each resistance-training workout needed to be an assault on our capacities and capabilities. They expected us to routinely and consistently exceed our limits. That is where all the gains and progress and muscle and power reside.

Rip a page from the playbook of the elite and expropriate the techniques, the tactics and their mental intensity. We too can storm the barricades of our limits in every training session, regardless our relative capacities on that day. We use a focused mindset to improve the quality of the individual training session. A rising tide lifts all boats: string together quality workouts like pearls on a strand and engineer the radical physical transformation we all seek.

2. CAPACITY IS A SHIFTING TARGET: ATTAINING "TRANSFORMATIVE CRITICAL MASS"

Regardless the resistance training tool used, success occurs when the human body is *forced* to reconfigure itself. We don't trick or fool the body into transforming; we force the body to morph, we force it to add more muscle and we force it to become stronger—all in direct response to the degree of effort exerted in our resistance training sessions.

To trigger the adaptive response and transform the body the athlete must approach, equal, or (ideally) exceed current exercise and strength capacity, in some way, shape, manner or fashion. Only by assaulting limits and capacities do we attain transformative critical mass. We understand that "capacity" is a floating target, one that changes daily and hourly, regardless, we seek to work up to capacity, wherever it might be on this day and time.

A man might be capable of bench pressing 300-pounds, exerting 100% of capacity on a good Saturday, might have a horrible fight with his wife or stress at the job and be off a full 15% on the following Saturday. On that day, an off day, 275-pounds might be all he is capable of. Regardless the actual finite capacity at any moment in time, our goal, our resistance mission, is to approach, equal or optimally exceed that capacity in some manner or fashion.

There are an infinite number of ways to express capacity and there are an equally infinite number of ways to express and then assault capacity. Let us take a look at some of the possibilities using our 300-pound bench presser. An elite athlete with a 300 x 1 100% max bench would have personal best performances in the different rep ranges: for example, a 300x1 bench presser could logically and realistically expect to have the following best "rep" lifts....

     300x1
     280x3
     260x5
     240x8
     220x10
     185x15

By establishing *benchmarks* in each of the different rep ranges, he can assault capacity in a variety of ways using the differing rep ranges as targets. Additionally, the attuned athlete understands that he might be having an off day and perhaps the 220 pounds he expected to rep for ten might stymie him, causing him to barely complete rep #7—this is fantastic in that he has hit 100% (or even a little more) killing himself (without breaking form) to lock out and rack the seventh excruciating rep: that rep was the transformative rep; that rep was the rep that released adrenaline and endorphins and cortisol and insulin and that rep was responsible for triggering the adaptive response. This man has made lemonade (gains) out of lemons (having an off day.)

Make no mistake about it, regardless if you are using a pair of dumbbells or a CrossCore®, pure physical effort, intensity, is the key to any and all muscle and power progress. The human body will not and does not favorably reconfigure itself in response to sub-maximal effort. Why would it? How could it? If sub-maximal exercise exertion generated actual results, ours would be a nation of Spartans instead of a nation of pathetic weaklings.

3. A MILE WIDE AND AN INCH DEEP... VOLUME VERSUS INTENSITY

Mainstream resistance training is overwhelmingly "volume based" whereas elite, hardcore strength training is overwhelmingly "intensity based." The elite understand that to achieve success, the key is not how much training you do but *how hard* you train. Mainstream resistance training experts and commercial personal trainers universally recommend a volume-based approach to resistance training, i.e., lots of exercises done with moderate to light poundage.

If all things were equal, insofar as results, volume-based resistance training would have a lot of advantages. Unfortunately, the inconvenient truth is the two approaches are not equal: low to moderate intensity progressive resistance regimens delivers subpar results. Without gut-busting physical effort, there is no improvement in performance, no increase in capacities and no favorable changes to the body. How could there be, why would there be? Where is the muscular stress needed to freak the body out and cause it to construct new muscle as a defensive measure?

We use the analogy that volume-based weight training is a mile wide and an inch deep whereas intensity-based weight training is an inch wide and a mile deep. The intensity-based trainer concentrates on a few select exercises and does them with bar-bending (relatively speaking) poundage. Reps are kept to ten or fewer; each successive week for the life of the periodized "cycle" the intensity-based trainer drives the training poundage upward, ever upward. We forcibly morph the body by demanding evermore of it.

Mainstream personal trainers feel this approach is "unsafe" and unnecessary: unsafe because the trainees routinely tax themselves and their abilities, unnecessary in that the mainstream, speaking with easy assurance of the blissfully ignorant, maintain that volume resistance training is equally effective and far safer. Wrong, wrong and wrong.

Orthodox mainstream personal trainers routinely have clients perform 12-20 different resistance exercises in a single session; resistance machines are preferentially used ("much safer") and the strategy is for the trainer to have the trainee plow through a dozen or more isolation exercises using low sets done for high reps. Light poundage is handled in sub-maximal, safe-as-milk fashion: fun, safe, sensible and sane, unfortunately the results are negligible. The cost-to-benefit ratio is badly out of balance, the results obtained from safe and sensible training are insignificant. The time and (sub-max) effort is not worth the trouble and expense.

Physical endeavors that are fun, safe, sensible and sane will not cause the human body to favorably reconfigure itself and we will not be satisfied with the results. Those that have actually successfully engineered a radical physical transformation can attest to the fact that a positively Herculean degree of effort is required, nothing of any physical consequence will occur in response to ease and sameness.

Elite Old School hardcore resistance champions uniformly favor intensity-based strength systems for one reason: they work. The results are positively spectacular and profound; time wise, intensity-based resistance training takes less cumulative weekly training time than a volume-based approach. While not time intense, the intensity-based system is extremely intense and physical: limits are breached every session.

 The intensity-based periodized training template would likely have a frequency of between two to four workouts per week. Session length is dependent on the strength levels of the athlete. Preplanned weekly training "micro" sessions are embedded into a larger, macro periodized game plan. Each cycle usually lasts from eight to 12 weeks. Each week, the athlete is expected to lift more poundage in training. Each successive week the poundage or reps are ratcheted upward. Physically and mentally, the elite strength athlete *attacks* each workout. We apply Old School strength tactics to this new tool, the CrossCore®, in an effort to elicit muscle and power gains from a portable training device. Our CrossCore® training efforts are intensity-based—an inch wide and a mile deep.

4. GRIND VERSUS EXPLOSIVENESS

Religious wars are often started over subtle, seemingly insignificant doctrinal differences of opinion. And so it is in the world of progressive resistance training. One au courant and unchallenged sacrosanct commandment of strength is that, regardless the tool, all repetitions in all progressive resistance exercises should be performed *explosively*.

The rationale is seductive and seemingly irrefutable: explosive reps convert into usable power, the kind of strength that can be applied on the ball field, battlefield, court, mat or track. Explosively dispatching the concentric, "loaded" phase of any rep on any lift is the accepted practice amongst the fitness intelligentsia.

The reverence for the explosive rep was not born in a vacuum. It was actually a strategy born to counter the thesis of the "slow and controlled" rep speed popularized by Nautilus and later super-slo advocates. Smart athlete-coaches like Fred "Dr. Squat" Hatfield and Michael Yeseis countered that the explosive rep was in itself an art and needed to be practiced. The Russians sought ways to increase explosive power for their armada of Olympic weightlifting champions. The Soviet Sport Review contained translations of Russian Olympic lifting strategies—explosiveness was the antithesis of the slow, controlled rep.

The Hegelian dialectic informs us that for every thesis an antithesis will eventually arise. Eventually that antithesis becomes staid and stale and becomes the new thesis—which in turn will give rise to a new antithesis, and so on and so on, ad infinitum. The ceaseless cycle continues ever onward. Meet the new boss, same as the old boss.

In the world of resistance training, explosive lifting came into vogue in the 1970s and was, at the time, the antithesis to the then accepted idea, the thesis, that control was preferred. Explosiveness was discouraged and denigrated by naysayers as an invitation to sloppiness. Explosiveness was dangerous, it was claimed, and exposed trainees to a much higher rate of injury.

Now in 2015 we have heretics, like us, that proffer up the idea that the time has come for a new antithesis—this in response to the sacrosanct doctrine of explosiveness; the explosive rep has become a stale cliché and while do not seek a return to the ridiculously slowed rep speeds that characterized the "slow reps" of yesteryear—instead we suggest the antithesis to the explosiveness: the "grind" rep.

Grind rep speed was born of injury. First introduced into elite progressive resistance circles by six-time Mr. Olympia, Dorian Yates after he experienced an injury in training doing explosive leg work, Yates was faced with a choice: slow his training rep speed or retire. Dorian slowed down—but just a tad—he "barely slowed" the rep speed. This is a subtle, critical point: Yates eliminated all momentum; he used continuous tension. His speed lowering and raising was identical: the same bar speed used on both concentric and eccentric.

Sometimes he would add pauses during the slowed rep to make the hard slow reps even harder. The mistake the super-slo advocates made was to slow the rep speed down way *too much*. The snail-pace they advocated resulted in the trainee being forced to use pathetic, pee-wee poundage. The super slo training became more an exercise in lactic acid tolerance than in muscle-building: super-slo was slow to produce any outstanding physical examples of people that had transformed as a result of slo-mo training.

Yates was a different kettle of fish and chips: Yates discovered that after becoming acclimatized to the new rep speed, he was able to reacquire 90% (or more in some exercises) of his best poundage when he had been lifting explosively. On many exercises, over time, Dorian was actually able to exceed his previous best efforts using explosive power. For example, his best explosive (touch-and-go) 45-degree incline barbell press was 405 for six reps. After fourteen months of grind work he hit 435 for six reps at which point, his training partner stepped in and administered two additional forced reps.

The purposefully slowed, yet not too slowed, rep speed has much to offer. Optimally we master all the rep speeds and periodically rotate them: when grind goes stale, embark on a period of explosive training and vice versa. Rep speeds are tactics, arrows for our resistance-training quiver; like hammers and screwdrivers. Does a hammer trump a screwdriver? Of course not—yet many in the fitness establishment seek to deify explosiveness. "Thou shalt have one God only!" They defend a rep speed as if it were the word of God.

While explosiveness is a fabulous attribute, it should not be our only attribute. Periodic rotation of rep speeds is both smart and productive. Bill Pearl, bodybuilding superstar and excellent amateur auto mechanic, once noted that "explosiveness is akin to horsepower; grind repping is akin to torque; optimally we want horsepower and torque." Those that practice one rep speed to the exclusion of the other will never realize their full physical potential.

We are resistance training explosiveness masters. However, our strength mentors made us first learn how to 'grind' a perfect rep, using a purposefully slowed rep speed. They made us grind with a full range-of-motion. Perhaps some pauses were thrown in to make the difficult even more so. Only after we young neophytes learned the proper techniques and only after these techniques had been ingrained using grind reps, did our iron masters instruct us on explosiveness. Exploding is easy once grinding is mastered.

Premature explosiveness, particularly for those that have not mastered the specified techniques, engenders sloppy inconsistency, every rep different than its predecessor, each rep differing in stroke length and degree of tension. Master the grind and come to explosiveness with ingrained techniques—and a high pain tolerance.

Grinding builds low-end pure bulldog torque; this type of strength is only built by muscling up rep after slowed rep. When grind-mastery is achieved, exploding is exhilarating, exciting and easy!

 Ancient power masters would require we rookie acolytes adhere to the gruesome grind strategy for months. It was an initial rite of passage that needed to be passed for admission into the tribe. The idea was to burn proper lifting technique into the acolytes' DNA. If they survived this trial-by-fire, they made the squad and earned the right to train with and under the Power Master. Pristine lifting technique was acquired and honed over the entire career of the lifter.

The hardcore, iron elite worshiped exercise technique and sought to improve upon current techniques. Better technique meant more efficient techniques and greater efficiency enabled evergreater poundage handling ability.

Grinding creates a degree of serious discomfort that intensifies as the set unfolds and progresses. Grinding is not a pleasant experience, yet one very real advantage to grinding is that less resistance is needed to invoke a huge muscular response. Grind speed makes "light weights heavy" whereas the rest of the fitness resistance universe is all about how to make heavy weights light.

Mainstream experts will tell you that exploding maximum poundage is a learned trait and that is correct. However, a man coming off two to three months of grind repping is the ideal explosive rep candidate. The man that has been forced to grind is the man most likely to correctly explode. The grind school graduate will have ingrained technique and consistency as he explodes. This creates the perfect storm for attaining all that explosive training has to offer. But we need graduate from resistance grind-college before we go to explosive grad school.

A half-century of high-level empirical experience tells us that allowing a novice to explode is an invitation to technical anarchy. Every rookie rep will be different and no groove pattern will be ingrained.

Once you have graduated grind boot camp, converting to explosiveness sends performance into the stratosphere. In our strength philosophy, explosiveness and grinds are not mutually exclusive. We are not dualistic, so the solution is not a question of one or the other. We need master both rep speeds and optimally we periodically need rotate these techniques.

Bottom line? When using the CrossCore®, mastery of the grind rep speed is a fundamental tenet: CrossCore® students need master the grind rep speed and avoid the tendency to become seduced by the far easier and far more fun explosive rep speed. We will explode soon enough. For now, let us first burn some technique into our DNA with grind.

SEEKING "THE FASTEST FORM OF SLOW"
THE CROSSCORE® MISSING PUZZLE PIECE: DORIAN YATES GIVES ME PERMISSION TO 'GRIND'

Back in the 1990s I was the top training article writer for the world's largest bodybuilding publication. During Dorian Yates' uninterrupted six-year reign, I had many conversations on and about training and nutrition with the Olympia terminator. I wrote numerous training articles about Yates and his methods for *Muscle & Fitness* magazine. He and I saw eye to eye on many, many aspects of progressive resistance training.

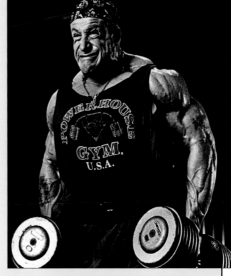

He was known for his shock-and-awe muscle mass and in person his sheer size was unbelievable. He stood 5-10 and in the off-season would work his bodyweight up to 300-pounds carrying no more than a 10% body fat percentile. He'd whittle this down to 260 sporting a 2% body fat percentile for the competition.

Here is how Yates looked weighing 300 pounds standing 5 foot 10 inches.

I remember interviewing him at a photo shoot that took place the morning after he'd stream-rolled his way to another title. One thing insiders knew about winning the Olympia: it was incredibly difficult to handle the aftermath... there was always a huge photo shoot scheduled for the winner the following morning. After the victory, the winner cannot celebrate: eating or drinking <u>anything</u> would cause swelling and distension and bloating and the winner would look smooth and subpar in the photos. So you go to bed hungry, not able to drink champagne or eat a steak—you need stay weak and emaciated one more excruciating day.

Yates was so ripped the Sunday morning after his Saturday night victory that as he sat and ate a dry bagel (he was carbing up immediately prior to the shoot) the muscles on his face were positively skeletal; his jaw and neck were so fat free that when he chewed it appeared his skin was translucent. All the tiny facial muscles we never see rippled as he chewed.

Yates had figured out a new way of training that enabled him to build more sheer muscle mass than any other IFBB pro bodybuilder. What set him apart from other big men was the degree of "condition" (low body fat) he was able to achieve. He was not only the biggest man onstage he was also the most ripped. This combination of size and condition allowed him to overcome his disproportional physique. True he had overwhelming mass and amazing degree of conditioning but he also had structural flaws: wide hips, smallish (for an IFBB pro) arms, a torn and disfigured bicep and a thick waist. His strengths overcame these shortcomings in the eyes of the judges.

I once wrote an article for M&F that compared the similarities in training between then Olympia dominator Yates, and the greatest powerlifter in history, Ed Coan. It was striking the degree of similarity of weight training used by both the world's best built man and the world's strongest man—each system was revolutionary within its respective universe and each man arrived at his system ignorant of and independent of the other's conclusions. Dorian was a hardcore "intensity" based trainer while the rest of the bodybuilding pros followed a classical high-volume, moderate intensity approach.

Yates was notoriously sullen with the press, yet he and I got on famously. Perhaps it was because unlike the journalism school geek squad of M&F and Flex staff writers, I was squatting 800 at the time and was the defending world master's powerlifting champion. He once said something that caught my deep attention and I quizzed him on this mercilessly: he told me that after he had injured himself (rather severely) by doing heavy and explosive back squats, he'd been forced to find tactical alternatives.

Explosive repping was out of the question. He'd been an explosive lifting exponent and advocate and now he was deprived of this fundamental training tactic: he could not lift explosively anymore: it was "slow down the rep speed" or retire. His solution was risky yet ingenious: he decided to stop performing his lifts explosively. From that point forward, he would "grind" his weights. His pushing and pulling speed would be even and smooth, both ascending and descending. Like a machine, he would rep with control and precision; he would remove every ounce of explosiveness from each and every rep.

He knew his ability to handle heavy weight would nosedive. He related that he had trepidation as he began experimenting. He discovered that slower, careful reps were creating some of the deepest muscular inroads he had ever experienced. He initially dropped poundage across the board: he had been handling 405 for six explosive reps in the 45-degree incline barbell press; this fell all the way down to 335 pounds for five reps, using the new purposefully slowed grind-speed.

What he told me was remarkable, "Initially my weights plummeted; it was depressing. Then an odd thing happened; over time, as I got more slower-rep sessions under my belt, my poundage starting climbing back up. I eventually got all my training weights back to pre-injury strength levels, when I was using explosion. I thought that quite unexpected." He also added 20 pounds of lean muscle to his already gargantuan body. The slow rep speed stimulated muscle fibers to a degree that momentum-tinged explosive reps couldn't match.

When the rep speed is slowed down and subjected to a full range of motion, muscle fibers are forced to contract and engage over every inch of every rep. I asked Dorian to define his slower, non-explosive rep speed. His answer was descriptive genius. "Barely slowed." If a rep is too slow, the amount of poundage plummets to an unacceptable degree. The idea was to "barely slow" the rep: it equated to the old iron axiom of "continuous tension." In the Old School continuous tension format, the ideal rep speed pushing or pulling, was the same, identical.

When using the CrossCore®, we seek to replicate classical barbell/dumbbell exercise techniques, seek to duplicate the physical intensity and we seek to duplicate the degree of muscular inroad achieved using classical barbell and dumbbell exercises. We strive to accomplish this in a wide variety of CrossCore® movements. We seek to consistently induce positive failure in ten or less reps. We found that a Yates' style Grind, barely slowed rep speed is ideal for use with the CrossCore®.

Does a muscle care what tool is used to induce the adaptive response? When I thought about creating intensity-amplifiers for the CrossCore®, Yates' post-injury rep speed strategy pushed its way to the forefront of my consciousness. Why not make the CrossCore® reps more difficult by slowing them down—but a la Yates, we barely slow the rep down. Too slow a rep speed destroys any semblance of poundage handling ability; we suggest that grind speed should be thought of as "the fastest form of slow."

5. INTENSITY AMPLIFIERS: MAKING THE DIFFICULT EVEN MORE DIFFICULT

We needed to make CrossCore® harder. When you use free weights, in order to make a movement harder, you throw more plates onto the bar or use heavier dumbbells. When an athlete uses the CrossCore®, to make what they are doing more difficult we increase the severity of the angle. For 90% of the world's population, the CrossCore® user can create an angle steep enough to bring themselves to positive failure in ten or fewer reps.

However, amongst the top 10%, the athletic elite, in many instances, we "run out of angle," using the CrossCore®. A man with a 200-pound overhead press is not likely to encounter positive failure in fewer than ten reps performing a set of regular speed front lateral raises no matter how steep the angle. So we "barely" slow that rep speed down. That in and of itself makes the exercise a good 25% harder.

We can add a pause and we can use a dramatically exaggerated range-of-motion, in conjunction with the steepest possible angle. If we are astute we can create payloads sufficient to cause strong men, elite athletes, to fail in a wide variety of CrossCore® exercises by rep ten. Tactics designed to make CrossCore® exercises more difficult are called "intensity amplifiers."

Intensity amplifiers are designed to increase the degree of difficulty; we seek ways to make pushing and pulling far more difficult—with the eternal caveat that we always maintain perfect exercise technique. We never compromise on using a full range of motion and we train with great psychological and physiological intensity.

Our single most heretical intensity amplifier is our idea of introducing *purposeful relaxation* into resistance training.

In mainstream resistance training, tension is King. Muscle tension is to be maintained throughout the entirety of every rep of every set; we attain and maintain muscle tension at all times at all costs. Trainees are taught to never lose tension, not even for a single instant. By maintaining continuous tension during every instant of every rep, maximum power is generated and maximum poundage can be handled.

The 'stretch-relax rep' is yet another intensity amplifier in the CrossCore® HardCore protocol. We learn to relax under a payload. The bodyweight of the CrossCore® user is used to create an "assisted stretch." From this relaxed stretch position, the CrossCore® user reengages the push or pull muscles and morphs from total relaxation to complete flexion by the conclusion of the rep.

This is unique: each and every rep starts with a stretched and relaxed muscle and then morphs into maximum muscular contraction. The severity of this type of rep needs to be experienced to be appreciated. The stretch & relax rep strategy, particularly when combined with grind, full ROM and perhaps some pauses, causes the degree of difficulty to skyrocket. The HardCore training protocol elevates the CrossCore® from superfluous toy to serious resistance training tool.

The CrossCore® expert combines gravity, bodyweight, and deep relaxation to geometrically increase payload. This type of training actually improves flexibility, keeps joints open and functioning, makes muscles pliable when relaxed and hard as wood when flexed. The stiffest of humans will be able to stretch a targeted muscle and then tax that muscle maximally—all in the space of a single rep. Over time, we increase the depth of the relaxation, the depth of the stretch and the degree of flexion.

1. On pushing exercises: relax and sink; allow bodyweight to stretch muscles at the beginning of each push rep

2. On pulling exercises: relax and sink; allow the bodyweight to stretch the muscles before beginning the pull phase of the rep

3. in each instance, complete relaxation is achieved by consciously and with great deliberation allowing bodyweight to forcibly elongate muscles

This strategy purposefully modulates (on every rep) between extremes: from total relaxation to total tension. If done dutifully, this approach works phenomenally well.

6. USING THE 3RD DIMENSION OF TENSION

The resistance training tools of choice (for elite athletes) are crude and cumbersome barbells and dumbbells. Free weights dig the deepest muscular inroad due in large part to their crude and cumbersome nature. Resistance machines are decidedly inferior because they eliminate the third dimension of tension, the need to control side-to-side movement. Free weight barbells and dumbbells *force* muscle stabilizers to spring into action in order to keep the barbell in the proper motor-pathway and adhering to the technical archetype of the selected exercise. Free weights force the athlete to adhere to a motor-pathway of their creation on every rep of every set.

Machines have "frozen" pathways. Machines are comfortable and easy to use and it is the comfort and ease that makes them decidedly inferior as muscle-building devices. Crude and cumbersome are far more beneficial for building muscle than ease and comfort. Progressive resistance exercise machines eliminate the need for stabilizers to control side-to-side movement. From a muscle-building/strength-infusing vantage point, machines cannot create the depth or degree of inroad attained using free-weights: it is a physiological impossibility.

The CrossCore®, in pulled-pin mode, causes muscle stabilizers to go crazy—and this is a fabulous attribute. The instability of the CrossCore® excites stabilizers to the same degree as handling a pair of dumbbells and for this reason the inherent instability of the pulled-pin CrossCore® trumps the inherent *stability* of a resistance machine.

TRAINING "THE CORE"

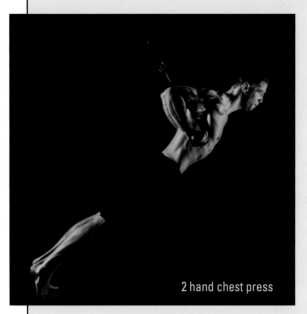

2 hand chest press

Many of the exercises in the CrossCore® HardCore protocol are performed in a plank position. This is not a passive body position. The legs, thighs, and glutes are maximally contracted. The abdominal muscles are braced, and consequently, the pelvis is locked onto the torso creating a neutral and stable spine.

The plank position required for CrossCore® HardCore training provides a platform to perform exercises such as the bicep curl, chest press, and row. Traditionally, these exercises have been artificially externally stabilized, using the preacher curl supports or any bench press. Using a body plank as a platform makes a CrossCore® HardCore press, curl, or row far more neurologically potent than the traditional version of each exercise. We seek self-generated "internal stabilization."

The added instability of pulled-pin mode makes maintaining the stabilized plank position much, much harder, requiring what Dr. Stuart McGill calls "anti-rotational" stabilization. So, in addition to stabilizing the spine in the sagittal plane (against flexion and extension) the pulled-pin mode requires a stabilized plank to resist spinal movement in the transverse plane against twisting and rotation. A CrossCore® HardCore one-arm bicep curl becomes a full body exercise.

The plank position and internal stabilization required for most CrossCore® HardCore exercises is itself an "intensity enhancer." We take a normal exercise and purposefully make it dramatically more taxing for the neuromuscular system. Enhancing the intensity of our exercises translates into more of an adaptive response (strength and hypertrophy) from the exercises.

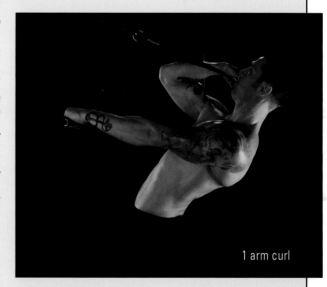

1 arm curl

7. IN SEARCH OF THE "BARELY COMPLETED" REP: FOOT SHUFFLE AND PAYLOAD

Because we are smart and subtle, we understand the need to create "struggle situations" in our progressive resistance training. One excellent intensity barometer is to continue a progressive resistance set until the athlete encounters the "barely completed" rep, the rep on which the trainee must struggle mightily in order to complete. As long as that rep occurs in less than ten reps we will create strength, power and muscle hypertrophy. More than tens reps and progressive resistance morphs into "strength endurance." Past 20 reps and we are into pure cardio modes.

We seek to create situations where we "create" barely completed reps on limit sets on a consistent basis, using our CrossCore® to mimic classic free-weight movements. By creating "struggle situations" with the CrossCore® we ensure that we reap the ample results associated with hardcore free weight training. The CrossCore® has some unique aspects that actually make the creation of struggle situations relatively easy—and in a surprising number of exercises.

1. The CrossCore® allows the user to *alter the payload mid-rep*. A simple foot adjustment is all that is needed to dramatically and instantaneously increase or decrease the amount of resistance the CrossCore® user is experiencing in real time, at that instant during the rep. This unique ability enables the skillful and astute CrossCore® user to modulate the payload to successfully create the highly desirable "barely completed" rep.

Optimally, our HardCore method enables you create an unending, never-ending series of barely completed final reps on the all important top sets of a wide range of beneficial exercises. A barely completed rep creates the type of inroad needed to reap real results. We seek out struggle and find that if we struggle with all our might, and if we barely manage by the skin of our teeth to finish a final rep, then you can expect to see real results for your efforts. The ability to vary the payload mid-rep on any rep is yet another fascinating attribute of the CrossCore®.

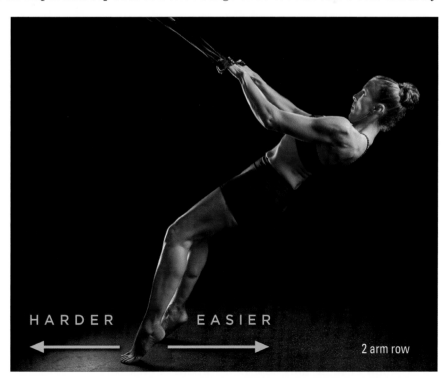

HARDER   EASIER

2 arm row

How would an experienced CrossCore® trainee successfully use the payload-altering "foot shuffle?" To increase or decrease resistance, we move our feet forward or backward, a matter of inches. The experienced CrossCore® user has "normal" distances established in each exercise—how far away do you stand from the CrossCore® anchor point, in each exercise, in order to elicit the proper resistance? What is the proper amount of angle needed to create sufficient resistance?

The exercise set starts with the athlete planked at the selected angle: the plank is locked out at knees, hips and shoulders; we are a rigid piece of meat to be raised and lowered in full rotational mode. The exercise commences and we use grind rep speed to bring us to just shy of positive failure in ten reps or less.

If after the first few reps the payload seems ridiculously light, shuffle forward or backward four to six inches. This small foot movement can increase resistance by 20-30%.

We seek titanic struggle. Sometimes the payload is too light and sometimes the payload is too heavy: the CrossCore® allows the trainee to make "in-flight" payload adjustments during the repetition. This might be unprecedented in the history of resistance training: imagine if we were able to "wish it" and barbells and dumbbells could become lighter or heavier. Would this not be revolutionary? We have that ability with the CrossCore®.

Very minor alterations in foot position—either toward the anchor or away from it—have a profound effect on payload: we alter intensity by modulating exercise intensity. Small foot changes have a dramatic impact. With time, this foot shuffle technique will become nearly automatic and enable the skillful CrossCore® user to land on any predetermined target repetition number—and just barely.

CROSSCORE® HARDCORE CHECKLIST

Before every set of every exercise create a plan of attack: select a technique then select a rep target and a rep speed....

1. Pick a target muscle or muscle group: select an exercise and select a technique for that exercise
2. Predetermine the repetition target: have a specific number of reps you intend on performing before you start any exercise
3. The CrossCore® HardCore protocol stresses repetitions in the five to ten rep range. We seek strength and maximum muscle hypertrophy
4. Adjust your payload resistance during the set. Seek to make the last repetition a barely completed repetition
5. Maintain pristine technique while exerting maximum intensity
6. Use a full range of motion on each repetition. If you cannot make a rep with a full range of motion, lighten the load or terminate the set

sagging

8. Use grind speed throughout the concentric (muscle shortening) and eccentric (muscle lengthening) phases of the exercise

9. We abide by the phrase, "barely slowed" to describe rep speed. Super-slow reps compromise poundage-handling ability to an unacceptable degree

10. Do not jerk or jolt to begin a rep. No bouncing or rebounding between reps. No contorting or breaking of posture when the push/pull becomes tough

11. Use pauses and stretch and relax to increase intensity

TECHNICAL NOTES

First, we need to reiterate our goal: we seek to maximize the adaptive response by engaging in resistance exercise using CrossCore® tool with HardCore protocols. The commandments assist in the achievement of our power and strength goal....

1. The five to ten repetition range creates strength when using the lower end of the rep range and hypertrophy is maximized using the upper end of the rep range. We are not training for muscular endurance.

2. The grind speed increases the amount of time under tension—a necessary component for hypertrophy—without veering into "super slow" rep speed territory. Too slow a rep speed dilutes physiological benefit.

3. We seek to eliminate momentum. When a muscle is using momentum, no muscle tension is generated. The barely slowed grind rep start builds "transitional strength."

4. Pausing reps builds "positional strength." Paused reps ensure we do not take advantage of rebound, the myotatic stretch reflex, that is used to accelerate the start of the subsequent repetition.

5. Emphasizing and controlling the eccentric (negative) phase is also a potent strength and hypertrophy inducer. Do not "throw away" valuable negative tension by letting gravity work in an uncontrolled manner.

6. The target of the "barely completed" final rep puts the muscle under maximum metabolic stress, another necessary component for a hypertrophic adaptive response.

The CrossCore® HardCore Checklist should be followed for every rep of every set of every exercise performed. Having said that as a generalized premise, advanced CrossCore® users have a training tactic that starts off a set using grind speed that adds "regular speed" reps when positive "grind failure" is reached. This subtle tactic enables the advanced trainee to continue the set "past failure." This tactic is the equivalent of a self-administered forced rep as used in classical free-weight training.

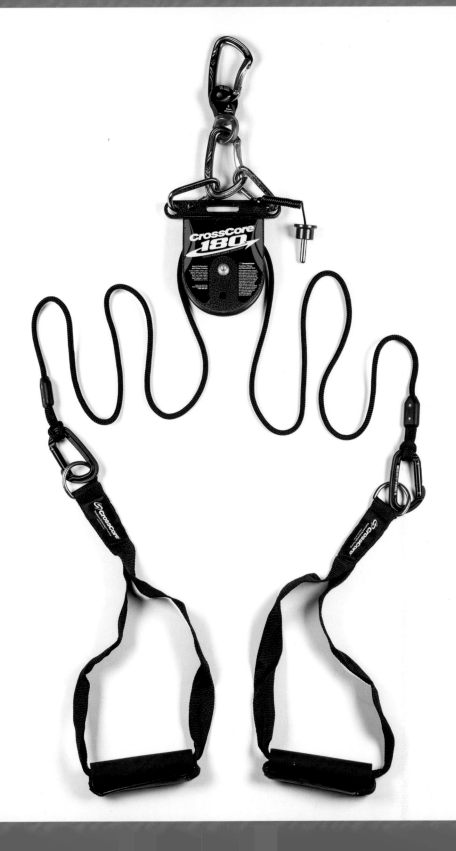

ANATOMY AND PHYSIOLOGY OF THE CROSSCORE®

SETTING UP THE CROSSCORE®

The CrossCore® can be attached to an anchor point allowing for either horizontal or vertical operation. We have divided the exercises in the CrossCore® HardCore protocols with respect to the horizontal or vertical operating mode. No matter the set-up configuration, ensure that the CrossCore® is securely anchored according to the instructions that ship with the device.

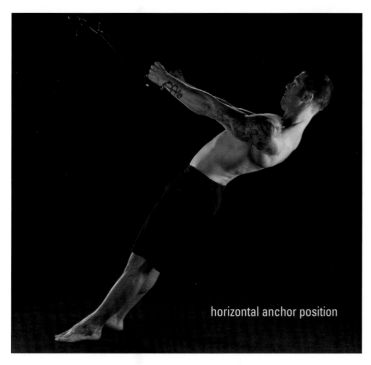

horizontal anchor position

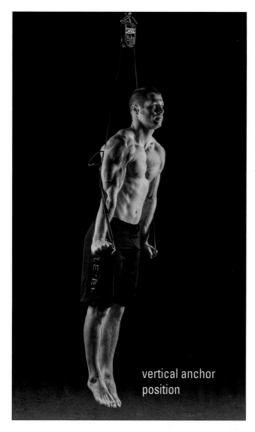

vertical anchor position

OPTIONAL SWIVEL MODIFICATION

We have added a swivel device to the CrossCore® setup for the CrossCore® HardCore protocols. The addition of the swivel allows for seamlessly switching between body positions without changing hand positions during exercises. For many of the exercises, the swivel also adds to the instability challenge of the device. Our protocols can be performed without the swivel, but we think it enhances use of the CrossCore®.

Note that the swivel device is not shipped with the standard CrossCore®, and is a modification not specifically endorsed by the manufacturer. Use this modification at your own risk, but by using the right hardware, the swivel can be incorporated safely. We use professional quality, locking carabiners and the rotor swivel made by Black Diamond, the rock climbing equipment company. Rock climbers trust their lives to this equipment while hanging hundreds of feet above the ground. The Black Diamond rotor swivel has a force capacity of over 5,800 lbs, satisfying our needs from a safety perspective. The configuration with the swivel and the CrossCore is pictured below:

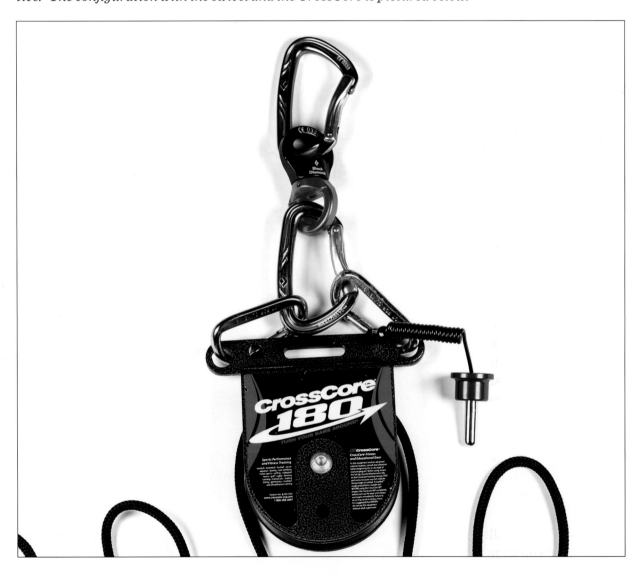

USING THE PIN

The CrossCore® patented pulley separates itself from other suspension trainers by use of a pulley that can be locked—or free for an extra level of challenging instability.

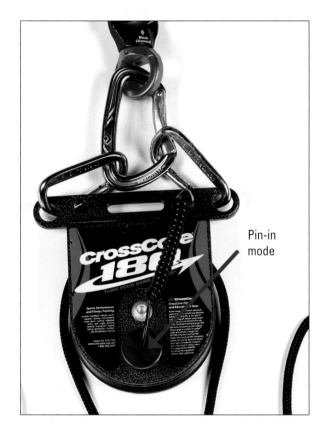

Pin-in mode

Pin-in mode locks the pulley and allows the user to push or pull with maximum stability. This mode is ideal for learning the techniques and ingraining the exaggerated range-of-motion favored by the CrossCore® HardCore protocols. Pin-in mode is the perfect way to get acquainted with new exercises that use very specific and demanding techniques before having to compensate for the highly unstable "pulled-pin" mode.

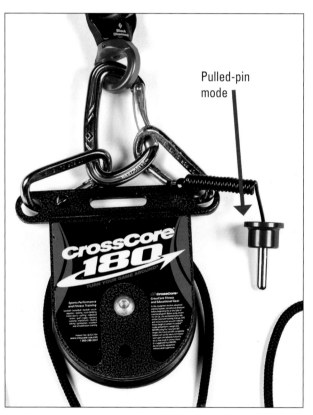

Pulled-pin mode

Pulled-pin mode unlocks the pulley and allows access to the uncharted hardcore exercise universe of rotational training. Literally a new dimension in exercise, the potential of rotational resistance training is just now being discovered. There is tremendous excitement among seasoned trainers, and now we have a way to apply significant resistance to an entirely new universe of exercise movements.

Pulled-pin mode also provides a highly unstable platform that multiplies the intensity and difficulty of even the most basic exercises. This results in a substantially greater neuromuscular impact for each exercise, as compared to its stabilized counterpart.

Pulled-pin mode allows for unilateral exercises that are almost impossible to effectively perform with other suspension training devices.

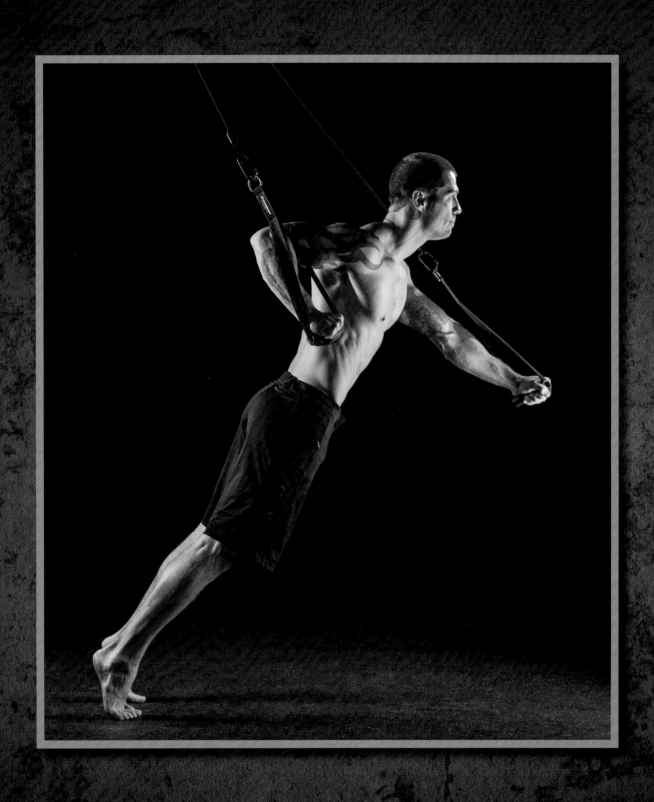

EXERCISE TECHNIQUES

HORIZONTAL ANCHOR EXERCISES

CHEST PRESS PROGRESSIONS

There are four iterations for CrossCore® HardCore chest presses.

1. Two-arm chest press with fixed pin
2. Two-arm chest press with pulled pin
3. One-arm chest press with pulled pin
4. Compound one-arm chest press with pulled pin

CHEST PRESS: TWO-ARM FIXED-PIN

1. Face away from the CrossCore® anchor point. Set your feet relatively wide
2. Grasp the handles and lower your body with tension as far as possible
3. The handles should be nestled on either side of your pectoral muscles
4. Now, still in the bottom position, exhale and relax, sink onto the handles
5. Release all tension in your chest and arms, allow bodyweight to stretch the chest and shoulder muscles
6. From this completely relaxed and stretched bottom position, re-engage the pectoral, deltoid, and tricep muscles and begin to push your planked body to lockout
7. Critical point: do not begin the push with a jolt or a fast and explosive start. We must discipline ourselves to use a "grind" rep speed
8. Grind rep speed is slow (not too slow; barely slowed) and consistently paced
9. Push inward (push the hands towards each other) as the difficulty increases—the natural inclination when pushing on the CrossCore® handles is to push outward
10. Achieve a full and complete lockout on every rep. At the conclusion of each chest press, flex the pectoral muscles and the triceps *hard*. Extreme flexion enhances results

11. The complete contraction at the top of each chest press rep is contrasted with the full relaxation and stretch at the bottom position of the rep. We alternate on every rep
12. Stretch-and-relax at the start of the rep; fully lock out each rep; use continuous tension, even and slowed rep speed, on both eccentric (lowering) and concentric (pushing)
13. The amount of resistance is increased by moving the feet closer to the anchor-point, or decreased (made easier) by stepping forward—away from the anchor point

TWO-ARM CHEST PRESS WITH PULLED PIN

One would think that there would be very little difference between a fixed-pin, two-arm chest press and a pulled-pin, two-arm chest press and one would be wrong: the degree of difficulty is increased significantly when both arms are forced to fight to create the equilibrium necessary to establish a stable push platform.

1. Assume the chest press position
2. Lower the body evenly and precisely; create tremendous tension as you lower
3. Relax in the bottom position, exhale, feel a stretch in the pecs and shoulders
4. Engage the pecs to begin to press. Do not jolt or jerk to start the press
5. Push yourself upwards smoothly with an even application of force
6. Your hands will tend to shake and vibrate as you push
7. Push with hands and arms aimed *inward*, do not allow the hands to flare outward
8. Complete lockout on every rep: straighten the elbows, flex the pecs and tris hard!
9. Make adjustments with your feet to obtain the optimal amount of resistance
10. Grip handles tightly to counter 'wobbliness.' We fight against instability

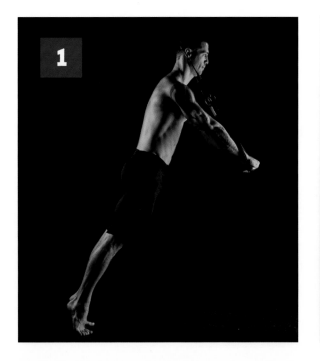 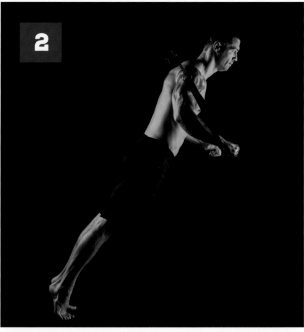

Pulled pin training allows the CrossCore® user access to the totally unique world of full rotational suspension training. The degree of instability created in full-rotational, pulled-pin mode causes muscle stabilizers to activate to a degree unobtainable by resistance machines and tools. Pulled-pin training can be used to create a dramatic muscular inroad that can rival gold standard dumbbells. Master the basic two-arm techniques before proceeding to the far more difficult single-arm exercises.

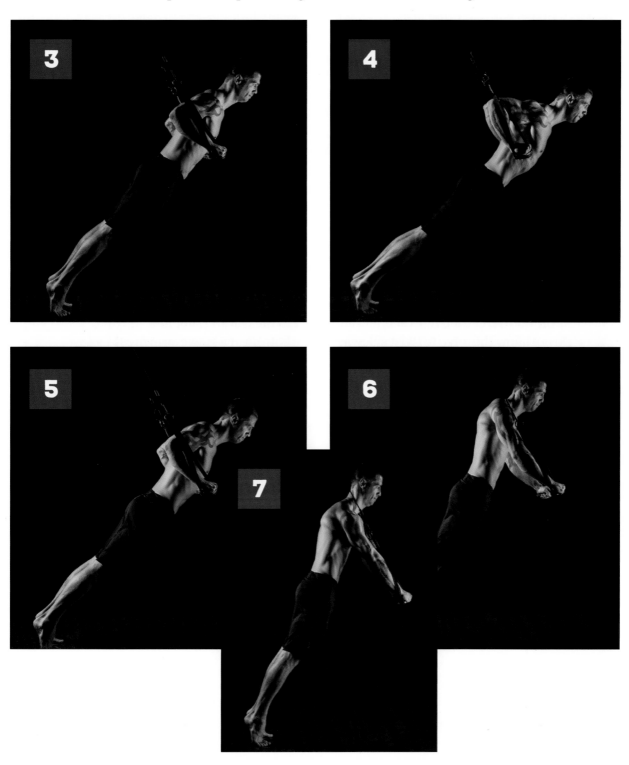

ONE-ARM CHEST PRESS WITH PULLED PIN

How do we amp up the resistance and the instability while chest pressing? We perform the single-arm chest press while keeping the non-pressing arm extended. This is a critical point: logic and ease would dictate that we "tuck" the free arm's fist (wrapped around the handle) tight against the chest as we push with the other arm. That would make pushing easier—to make pressing more difficult, always our goal, we keep the non-working arm extended. In order to maximize instability, we will keep the non-pushing arm extended throughout the set. This will feel awkward initially (and maybe forever.) We *force* static stabilizers of the extended arm into action.

With one-arm extended and rigid, break the elbow and begin lowering the torso with other arm. At the bottom of each single-arm chest press rep, relax and sink and stretch the pec and shoulder of the pressing arm. Reengage and grind the rep to lockout. Avoid the tendency to "open up" and turn sideways at the bottom of each rep. In the bottommost position, relax, lose muscular tension *on that side only.* Half the body will stay rigid and tensed, the other half will relax and sink into the pressing arm handle before beginning the push phase chest.

1. Assume the classic chest press stance
2. With both arms extended, "pull" one-arm towards the chest
3. Use the slowed and precise lowering for the pressing arm
4. The stabilizing arm remains extended and contracted throughout the set
5. At the bottom of each rep, relax and sink, stretch the pec and shoulder
6. Do not allow the torso to twist sideways in the bottom of a single-arm press
7. Complete all reps on one-arm before beginning with the other arm

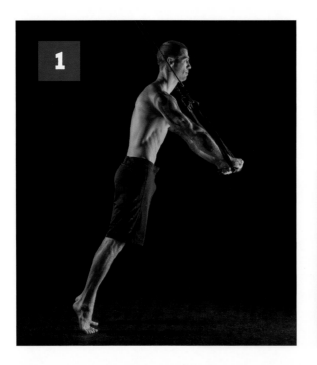
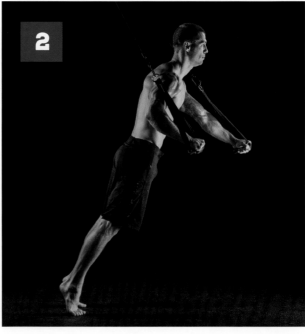

8. Do not jolt, jerk, twist or contort to finish a rep
9. On the final rep for the first arm, hold the final lockout position
10. Lower the "fresh" arm and repeat the procedure
11. Use your intuition to increase or decrease the resistance, rep by rep

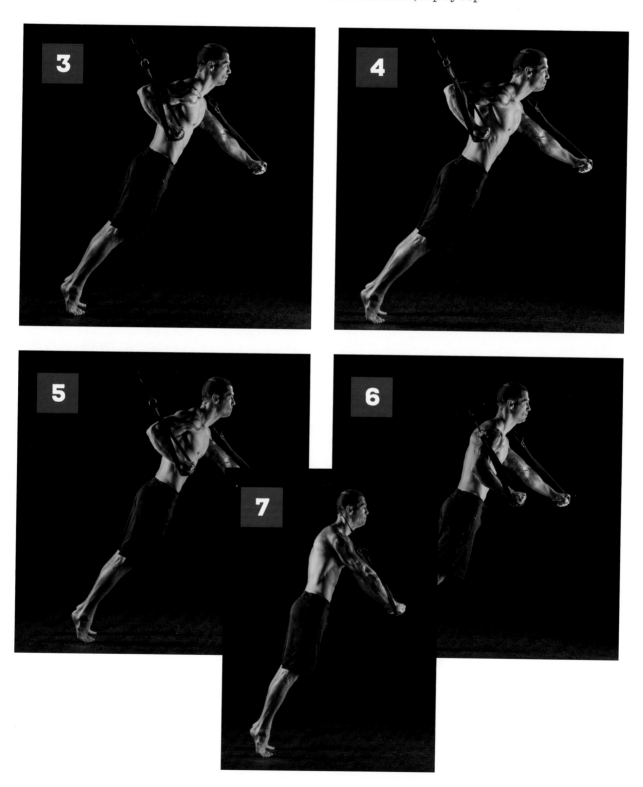

ROTATIONAL STRENGTH

When engaging in resistance training we usually work with a tool or implement in a straight line. If the tool is a barbell, dumbbell or kettlebell, nearly all of our resistance-training efforts will be pushed, pulled, raised, or lowered, in a straight line. The rep goes up and then it comes down. A few minor exercises use a curved motor-pathway (curls, tricep extensions, leg curls), but we mostly train strength in straight lines.

Straight-line resistance training is fantastic for loading a targeted muscle, terrific for intensely stimulating muscle fibers, and terrific for developing hellacious strength... but is that all there is?

We actually want more—we want all the "up-and-down" benefits from straight-line training PLUS we want another type of strength—rotational strength.

1. We seek dynamic rotational strength, the kind needed to fling a discus, perform the Fosbury flop or punch and kick with lightning speed and sledgehammer power. How can we obtain rotational strength if we don't train for it? How can up-and-down straight-line training give us the rotational force we need to further our athletic pursuits? We now have a tool and protocol specifically suited to building dynamic rotational strength: the CrossCore®.

The CrossCore®, used with HardCore protocols is ideal for creating, improving and increasing a trainee's rotational strength. We will go a step further and say that there is no finer fitness tool on the market for developing rotational strength than a properly used CrossCore®.

The potential turns into reality when the CrossCore® user implements the CrossCore® HardCore strategies and protocols we designed to accompany this amazing tool. Consistent wrestling with a CrossCore® is the best way to build, develop and increase your current quota of rotational strength.

The movements need be technically correct, and performed on a systematic basis with the requisite degree of intensity and effort. That said, if you obey the rules, and are consistent, your usable rotational strength can be increased by 50% in four weeks. That's no joke.

Think of an athletic motion like swinging a bat, throwing a ball, throwing a punch, or kicking a ball—the one component that links all these activities is rotation. Unbeknownst to you, you are most likely weak in rotational strength. We can fill in this "blank spot" by using the CrossCore® in full rotational (pulled-pin) mode.

We can train the body to exert power and torque as it rotates through time and space; we can train the body to create flow by synchronizing positional strength and transitional strength to create rotational strength. We can train the body by ingraining beneficial neurological pathways. Rotational capability and capacity cannot help but be improved through the systematic use of the CrossCore®. Improved rotational strength will allow you to move more efficiently, generate more force, and become a better athlete, fighter or soldier.

Positional and *Transitional* strength are important aspects of the complete strength spectrum. Rotational strength is equally important and of the three, might be *the most important* type of strength to possess for enhancing athletic performance.

Examples of rotational strength in action abound: think of the "shoulder throw" in Judo or MMA. Massive rotational forces are generated as the athlete enters the opponent's defensive zone, sets up and explosively executes the rotational throw. Optimally, this happens effectively with snap, power and the release of tremendous coiled energy.

Learning to generate force is a skill dichotomy: generating significant force is both a basic skill and an extremely advanced skill. Some of us are inherently adept at generating rotational strength and some of us are inherently impaired.

One of the unique training aspects of the CrossCore® is that employing it allows the user, regardless if you are adept or inept, to train loaded movements with rotation and in doing so systematically improve rotational strength, regardless the ability or inability of the trainee.

Expert use of the CrossCore®, in full rotational mode, creates *real* training. Real training means difficult rotations performed under stress, well beyond maximum effort and all done in a rotational format. This is tough stuff, not the light and easy rotations associated with say a Zumba dance move sequence.

We need to put the athlete under an intense rotational load; then teach them the most efficient way to transfer loads and generate force while powering through to completion. The adaptive response generated using this unique tool in rotational fashion is unprecedented and is nothing short of revolutionary.

Performed correctly, CrossCore® HardCore rotational protocols are extremely demanding—physically, psychologically and neurologically.

Consistent rotational training teaches the athlete to become adept at force generation, from the ground to the extremities. We can use the CrossCore® to build exceptional awareness of our body in motion.

We need to make our transitions strong and the CrossCore® is an ideal tool for the job. We need to improve rotational strength and fill in power gaps and strength weak spots. The alternating rotational chest press is an ideal way to start exploring rotational strength training.

ALTERNATING ROTATIONAL CHEST PRESS

The rotational press amplifies the chest press range-of-motion and in doing so engages not only the pectoral muscles but the front, rear and side deltoids, the rhomboids and teres, all must combine and synchronize movement in the sagittal and transverse planes to power this complex exercise from start to finish. This particular technique allows us to work in a rotational fashion unique to the CrossCore®.

1. CrossCore® is in pulled-pin configuration, assume chest press start position
2. Both arms are locked out
3. Lower yourself as if you were performing a one-arm chest press
4. At the bottom, relax and feel a stretch in the pectoral muscles
5. Turn the torso slowly to the right or left (depending on which arm is used)
6. Keep the fist tucked next to the pec as you turn slowly towards the rear
7. Allow your hand to move behind the torso
8. Allow the pushing arm to extend straight behind the body
9. At the low point, one-arm remains straight and in front
10. At the low point, one-arm is straight and behind the body

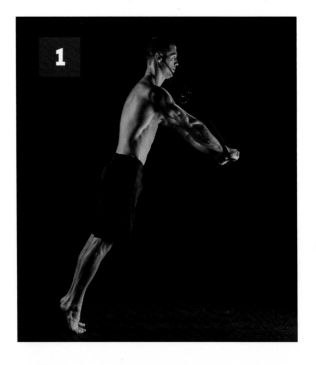
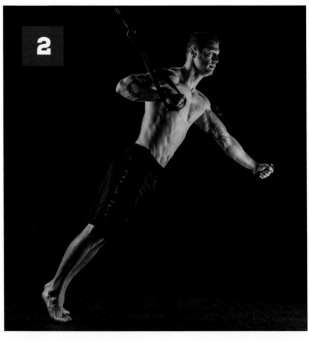

11. The torso should remain in a "plank" position as it turns sideways
12. The feet rotate towards the "open" side but do not change position
13. The torso and arms now form a graceful and powerful "T"
14. Next we reverse: pull the back arm (fully extended) towards the torso
15. Lead with the fist: the athlete powers his bodyweight in a rotational fashion
16. The critical point: "turning over the fist" both on lowering and raising
17. The rear arm is pulled into the torso, with power
18. The fist turns over; now push the fist to lockout
19. When pulling the behind–the-body arm towards the torso, mimic a "flye" exercise
20. The flye tension reaches maximum difficulty just as the fist is turning over

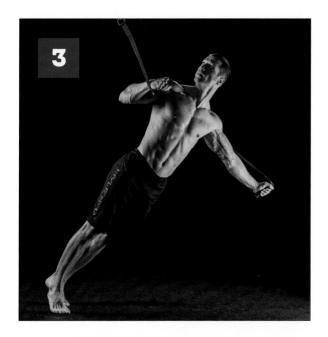
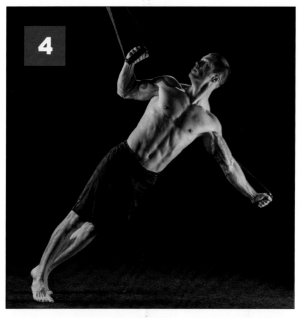
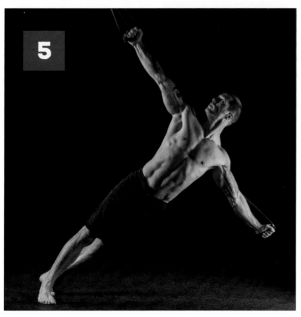
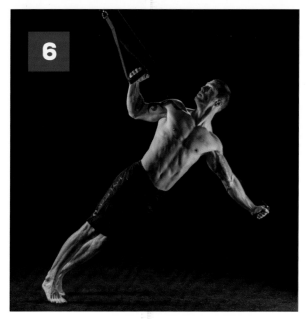

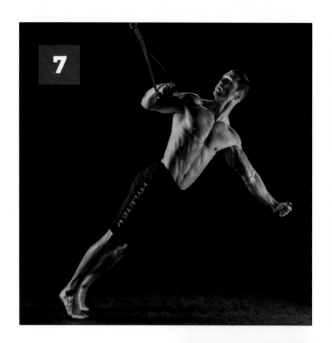

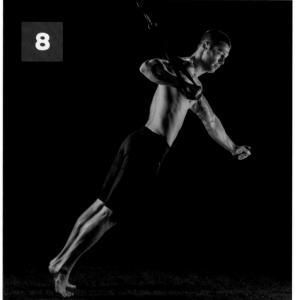

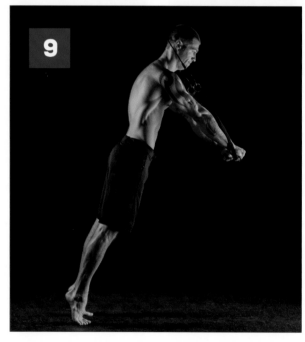

ROW PROGRESSIONS

The row is the opposite of the chest press. Properly performed, rows build posterior back muscle and will balance out the average gym-rat's forward sloping and rounded shoulders—the result of too much bench-pressing without training the complimentary muscles of the upper back. The latissimus dorsi are the most underused muscles on the human body, because of their unique function: they are used to pull the arms in towards the upper torso. We don't have much need for tasks that require this type of pulling and minor inward pulling is accomplished by the biceps.

Because of their underutilization, when we are able to institute a regimen of rowing that actually makes the mind/lat connection, the "lats" come up fast. The mind/muscle connection requires that we row with our lats and not our biceps. Proper CrossCore® rowing will build and strengthen all the muscles of the mid and upper back: the rhomboids, posterior deltoids, middle trapezius, along with the latisimus dorsi muscles.

MEDICAL NOTE:

Overdeveloped pectoral muscles (pushing) and weak pulling muscles can lead to a muscle imbalance called *"Upper Crossed Syndrome"* (UCS) first described by famed Czech physician Vladimir Janda. UCS is the underlying cause of many neck and shoulder injuries in modern society.

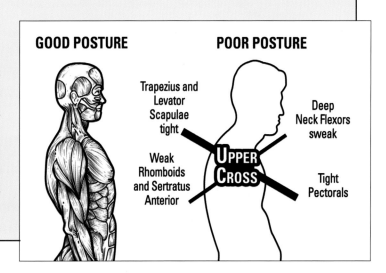

When properly stimulated with rowing exercises, the previously underutilized middle and upper back muscles grow and strengthen dramatically. Unfortunately, few people are able to make the mind-muscle connection with their back muscles and end up rowing with their arms. The biceps love to row. We used to have a saying, "Show me a man with terrific biceps and I'll show you a man with subpar lats." And conversely, show me a man with incredible lats and I will show you a man with subpar biceps.

In order to obtain the desired benefit from our rowing, we need to stop the biceps from doing the work. The best way to take the biceps out of the rowing is to simply place the thumbs on top of the CrossCore® handles when we row. Normally, we form fists around the CrossCore® handles. But for rowing, don't grip the handles in the conventional way. The four fingers of each hand will encircle the CrossCore® grips—make sure the leather hand strap is secured tightly across the top of each fist—and the thumbs do not circle and grip the handle. Lay the thumbs atop. Once the thumbs are removed from the grip, the biceps are prevented from assisting the lats in the pull.

The key to successful rowing is to make the back do the work of pulling. Check to make sure that the back is engaging and that the biceps stay relaxed. Just as the biceps will contract on every rep of a perfect curl, the back muscles should contract on every rep of every row. Many folks have "back amnesia" and struggle to get the lat muscles to fire. You can overcome this issue with conscious effort and close attention on each and every rep. The key is awareness: either your back muscles contract in reaction to pulling—or they do not.

THE ROW PROGRESSIONS:

1.   Two-arm row with fixed pin
2.   Two-arm row with pulled pin
3.   One-arm alternating row with pulled pin
4.   Rotational extended row

TWO-ARM ROW WITH FIXED PIN

The best and easiest way to learn how to row is to start with the CrossCore® in both hands with the fixed pin. This will cut the variables to a minimum and allow the user to really concentrate on engaging the back.

1.   Face the CrossCore® and grasp the handles
2.   Insert your hands under the straps, and pull the straps tight
3.   Place your thumbs on top of the handles
4.   While maintaining a straight "planked" torso, lower yourself backward
5.   Relax at the bottom and feel your back muscles stretch
6.   Turn your wrists upward one-half turn to engage back before pulling
7.   Begin the pull with a smooth application of power
8.   Use the grind rep speed
9.   Pull with "the elbows", not the arms
10.   Pull until the elbows are behind the torso
11.   Fists should end up next to the lower pecs
12.   Contract the lats hard all during the rep
13.   Lower with great tension and precision
14.   Relax in the bottom position before beginning the next rep

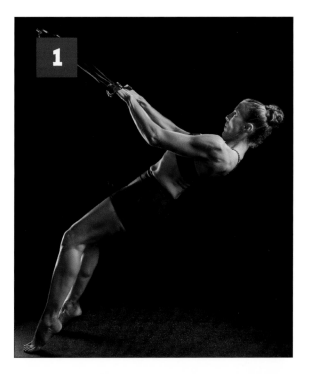

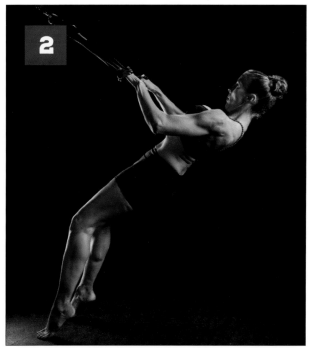

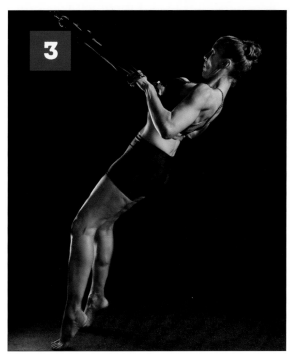

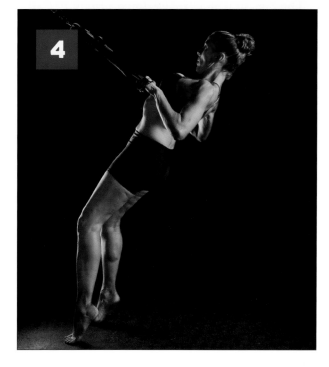

TWO-ARM ROW WITH PULLED PIN

CrossCore® users are shocked at how much more difficult it is to perform a two-arm row with the pin pulled as opposed to the same exercise done with fixed pin. The degree of difficulty is much higher when instability is introduced.

1. Use the same set up procedure as the two-arm fixed-pin row
2. Make the mind/muscle connection with the lats
3. Back pull the payload; avoid pulling with the biceps
4. Experiment with steeper angles to increase resistance
5. Do not let technique disintegrate when a rep becomes difficult
6. Better to fail than break technique in order to complete a rep
7. Decrease the row's resistance by inching backward during or between reps
8. If needed, increase the resistance by inching forward between reps

ONE-ARM ROW WITH PULLED PIN

The fastest way to make a two-arm pulled-pin row more difficult is to perform it with one-arm. First familiarize yourself with the two-arm row and make sure you can make the mind/muscle connection before trying the single-arm row.

1. To begin the one-arm row, lay back in the plank position
2. Engage the lats at the start of the pull
3. Begin with the weaker arm
4. Engage the lat as you begin pulling
5. Pull using the grind rep speed
6. A smooth, even and powerful pull ends with the fist at the armpit
7. Do not let the torso rotate to the "open side" at the end of the pull
8. Lower with tension
9. Begin pulling with the strong arm, ending at the arm pit
10. On each arm, the elbow should end up behind the torso
11. Do not rotate the torso at the end of the move

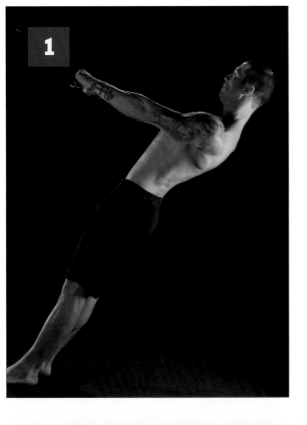

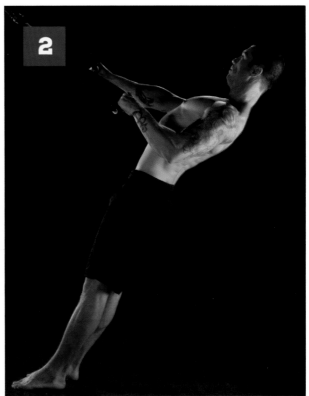

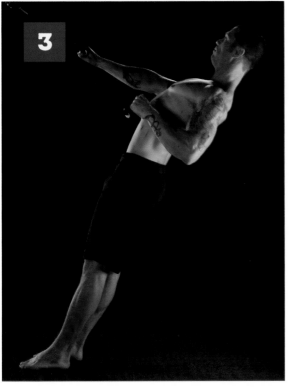

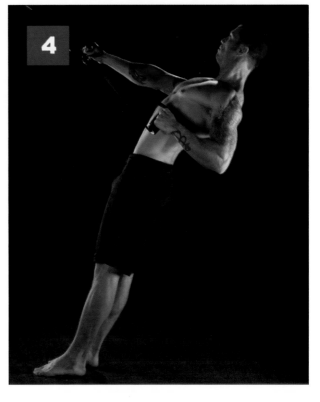

ROTATIONAL EXTENDED ROW

Once you are familiar with the two-arm row with pulled-pin, once you have spent some time mastering the one-arm row with pulled pin, you should be ready to move on to the most difficult and complex row: the rotational extended row. This is an extremely advanced row and should only be attempted once you have a solid foundation in the two-arm and one-arm rows.

1. To begin the rotational extended row, lie back in a plank position
2. With the handles held palm-down, imagine "breaking the bar" to create tension in the lats and torso. This will establish a strong and stable base for initiating the row

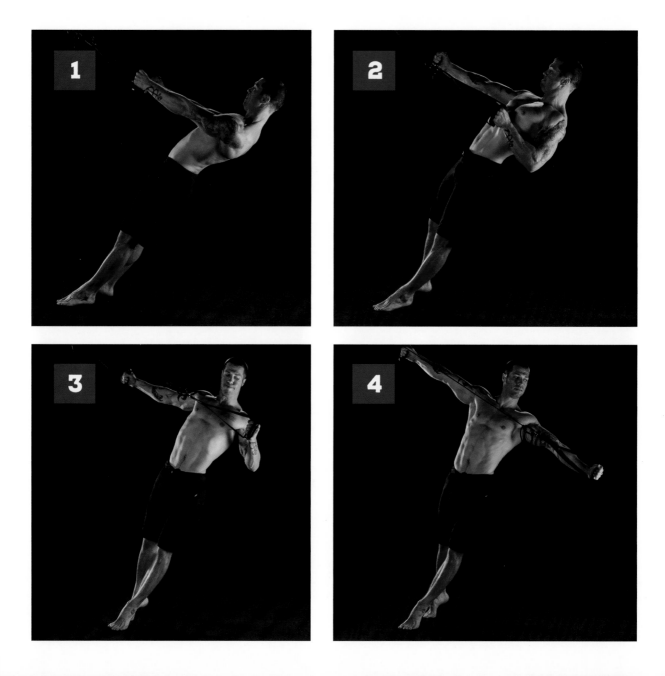

3. Start the row with the weaker arm, firmly engaging the lats and keeping the elbow close to the torso
4. Pull using the grind rep speed throughout the movement and all transitions
5. When the fist meets the armpit, continue to pull the elbow back
6. Transition into pressing the handle away from the body
7. Allow the torso to rotate under control, and follow the fist with your eyes
8. During the rotation, allow the feet to rotate
9. Maintain a solid base and maintain control
10. Continuing pressing until the elbow is fully locked
11. Reverse the process by using a "mirror image" motor-pathway reversal

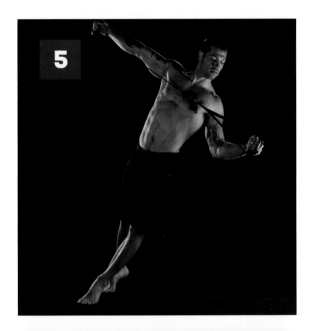

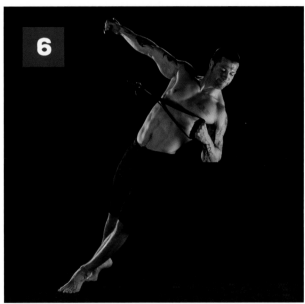

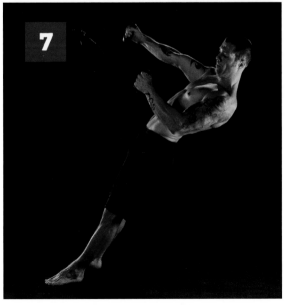

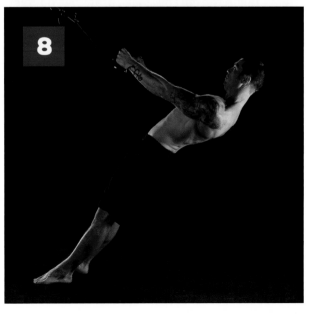

CURL PROGRESSIONS

For a variety of reasons, bicep training, curling and curl variations are perhaps the easiest CrossCore® exercises to learn. The technical ease and mechanical simplicity of curling makes it the most easily understandable of all the CrossCore® HardCore progressive resistance training exercises. It is very natural to face a CrossCore®, lie back in a plank position, and then perform a perfect set of grind-style bicep curls. The muscular response derived from curling while using the CrossCore® HardCore strategies can replicate the degree of inroad achieved using a pair of dumbbells.

Trainees should begin curling using the fixed-pin, two-arm bicep curl. Become familiar with the tool, the technique and the strategy and establish the always-important mind/muscle connection. This last point is critical: making the mind/muscle connection is the essence of CrossCore® HardCore. How do you know you have successfully made the mind/muscle connection? Simple, you should feel the targeted muscle "working" (contracting) in real time. The bicep curl performed on the CrossCore® and utilizing HardCore protocols is a prime example of how "intensity amplifiers" can be utilized to geometrically increase results.

TWO-ARM BICEP CURL WITH FIXED PIN

The goal is to meld technique with "feel" (mind/muscle) over a full and complete range-of-motion. Half reps and partial reps will only deliver half and partial results.

1. Face the CrossCore® pulley; assume a "mild" planked position at a high angle
2. Lay back as far as possible with palms facing upward
3. Both arms are straight and relaxed
4. Begin the curl by *slowly* drawing your clenched fists towards your face
5. Do not jolt or jerk to begin the movement
6. Raise your elbows as you curl, slowly moving into shoulder flexion
7. The elbows will want to drop as you curl—resist that tendency
8. Do not allow the elbows to flare outward as you curl
9. As the curl proceeds, turn the wrist and hands outward (supination)
10. Use the grind (slowed down) speed on both concentric and eccentric phases
11. At the end of the two-arm curl, your fists should be clenched by your face
12. Flex the biceps *hard* at the top of the curl
13. Begin lowering, fighting the lowering with biceps flexed
14. Maintain a crisp plank position throughout, do not sag
15. At the very bottom of the curl, *relax* the biceps and lose all arm tension
16. From complete arm relaxation, reengage the biceps and begin the next rep
17. Make adjustments to the resistance
18. To lighten the load, move forward, for a greater challenge, move back

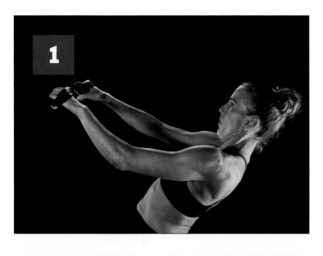

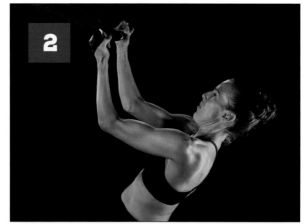

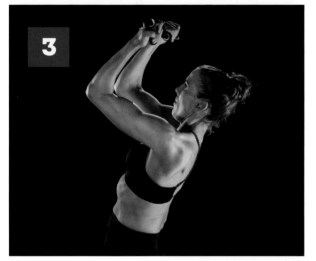

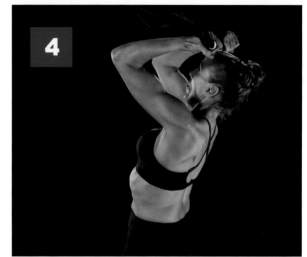

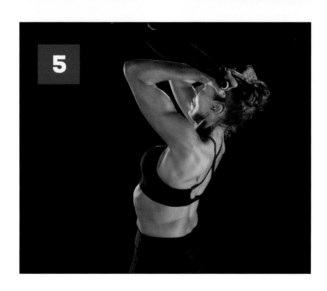

INCREASING TIME UNDER (EXTREME) TENSION INCREASES RESULTS

We create tremendous resistance/intensity during the curl by maintaining intense internal stabilization while in the plank position. HardCore protocols engage the biceps in a way seldom if ever seen in traditional arm training.

Most of us are aware that the main function of the biceps is to flex the arm at the elbow. The two heads of the bicep muscle attach to separate points on the scapula and assist in shoulder flexion. The CrossCore® HardCore biceps curl technique calls for lifting your elbows as you perform the curl. This technical mandate requires the biceps to assist the anterior deltoid in shoulder flexion. This is why our bicep curl technique maximally stimulates the biceps, amplifying the adaptive response and hypertrophy. We curl in such a way as to make curling more difficult: difficulty in resistance training equates to results.

Once the trainee can isolate the biceps with the two-arm curl in fixed-pin position, it is natural and appropriate to move to the two-arm curl using pulled-pin mode. Master these "unstable curls": then graduate into the various one-arm curl variations. All curl variations build on the techniques first developed with fixed-pin, two-arm curling. Avoid the temptation to skip ahead to the more advanced curling variants: master the preliminaries and solidify technique before tackling the tricky one-arm variations. Drill technique! Better to do five controlled, focused, perfect reps than a dozen sloppy, inconsistent "fun" reps.

TWO-ARM BICEP CURL WITH PULLED PIN

Curling difficulty is amplified to a significant degree by pulling the CrossCore® pin and introducing an element of instability. Unlike many other exercises, the difference between pin-in, two-arm curling and pulled-pin, two-arm curling is relatively minor. The pulled-pin curl is more difficult, but not to the same dramatic degree as with a chest press or dip.

ONE-ARM BICEP CURL WITH PULLED PIN

The degree of difficulty increases significantly when we shift from two-arm curling to single-arm curling. For starters, the resistance will need to be reduced by inching your feet forward towards the anchor-point. While learning the one-arm curl, take your time and avoid the common mistake of using too steep an angle or slowing curl speed down too much. If the resistance is too much too soon, you will twist, contort and break form to complete the movement. Start off light and easy. Smooth and machine-like curling uses a full and complete range-of-motion. Add resistance once perfect technique is dialed in.

1. Adhere to all the bullet-points outlined in the two-arm pin-in curl
2. Begin the one-arm curl in the same way as the two-arm bicep curl
3. The body is in a plank position with arms straight and biceps relaxed
4. Start the one-arm curl with the weaker arm
5. Grind upward without jolting, speeding up or contorting
6. The non-curling arm stays straight while the active arm curls
7. Simultaneously raise the elbow of the working arm as you curl
8. At the top of the rep, flex the bicep hard
9. Lower yourself with precision, while "feeling" every inch of the descent
10. "Rep out" on one-arm before switching, do not alternate arms on each rep
11. Repeat the procedure using the stronger arm
12. To build the mind/muscle connection, feel each bicep work in real time

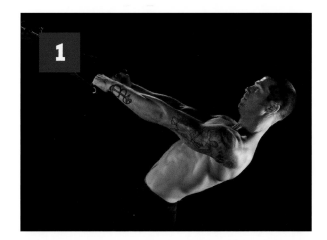
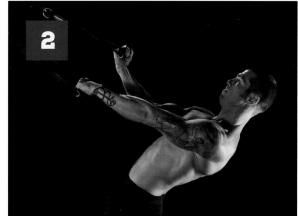
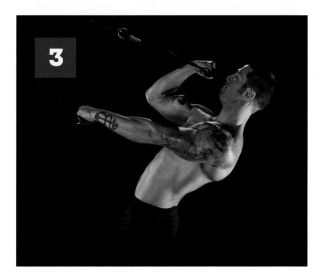
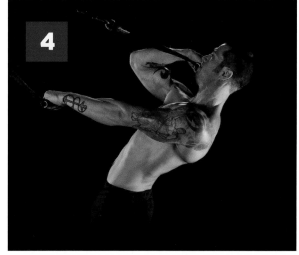

ADVANCED BICEP CURLING

There are countless ways to amp-up the already difficult one-arm curl, taking curling into the difficulty stratosphere. Our "intensity amplification" strategies have stopped some of the strongest of men in the world (men capable of strict barbell curls with 200 pounds) in less than ten reps.

1. Extreme angles: shorten the strap, place your feet closer to the anchor
2. Weighted vest: wear a weight vest loaded with an extra 5-50 pounds
3. Partner-resisted: a training partner places a resisting hand on the trainee's chest
4. Partner-assisted: go to positive failure, partner then provides assistance for forced reps
5. Extended sets: rep out on each arm, then immediately rep out with both arms
6. Drop sets: successive sets of non-stop curls, on each set reduce the resistance by changing the angle

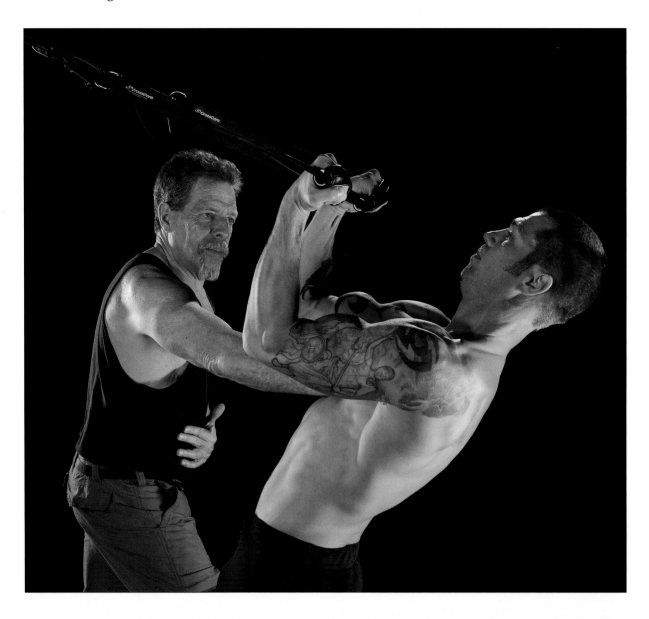

TRICEPS PRESS PROGRESSIONS

The triceps constitute 65% of the upper arm. Compared to the smaller and weaker bicep muscles, the triceps are far stronger, larger, more powerful and used much more in our daily lives. As the name implies, the triceps consist of three separate contiguous muscles whose function is to push away from the body. Old school barbell and dumbbell training recognizes five classic triceps exercises, and each has a very specific technique. The triceps can be attacked while lying, sitting, or standing—and from a variety of angles. The CrossCore® is particularly adept at replicating the classic dumbbell one and two-arm *triceps extension*. Most expert free weight trainers recognize extensions (and dips—another exercise the CrossCore® can replicate) as the finest of all triceps exercises.

The triceps extension is traditionally performed using a narrow grip with the barbell, dumbbell or machine handles held in the hands with palms facing away. The upper arm is stabilized from the chosen posture and the mission is to straighten the acute angle formed by the forearm and upper arm. As long as the upper arm is frozen, you may push while seated, standing, lying or inclined. Only the forearms move to push the weight to lockout. With triceps exercises, lockout is always considered to occur when the arms are straightened—hard.

Both the pushing concentric phase, and eccentric retracting phase, can be performed at one of three distinct speeds: purposefully slowed, normal (regular), and purposefully accelerated. Each has a different muscular effect.

Regardless which tool is used, technique must be consistent. One technical mistake we continually see in triceps training is when a trainee allows their elbows to flare out to the side as the push phase is completed. This "trick" effectively reduces the resistance when passing through the sticking point. While this tactic might allow you to handle more reps of greater resistance, it is unacceptable behavior if you want to build triceps and increase arm strength. The diligent CrossCore® user makes it a point to fight through the sticking points, which are where the power, strength and size gains reside. We do not avoid sticking points; we seek them out and embrace them.

Using the CrossCore®, an athlete intent on training the triceps can replicate the classic gold standard: dumbbell triceps extensions., The CrossCore® also allows the user to perform the venerable and highly effective dip. An infinite variety of exercise possibilities exist within these two classic triceps movements. Use tension, control, mindfulness and a full range-of-motion. Find and fight though sticking points.

TWO-ARM TRICEPS PRESS

Many individuals find triceps presses are somewhat awkward. Very few things in life require dropping a weight behind our heads, or lowering a weight to our faces while using a narrow grip that provides very little leverage. Over time, and assuming technique is correct, strength and size gains come quickly. Once you have developed solid technique with the two hand fixed-pin setup, pull the pin and perform the identical exercise. By simply pulling the pin, we introduce a mild degree of instability that makes pushing far more difficult. Become adept at two-hand, fixed-pin and two-hand, pulled-pin triceps presses before trying the exponentially more difficult one-arm triceps press.

1. Face away from the CrossCore® anchor point. Set your feet relatively wide
2. Grasp the handles and straighten both arms until they are locked
3. Knees are bent and hips flexed
4. The body from glutes to fists are now parallel to the ground
5. Maintain the parallel body position
6. Start the movement by bending your elbows
7. Lower with muscular tension until your elbows are maximally flexed
8. At the bottom of the movement, handles are nestled on each side of the head
9. Exhale and relax onto the handles; this "pre-stretches" the triceps
10. Re-engage the triceps and methodically push to open the elbow angle
11. Maintain a body position parallel to the ground
12. Do not let your upper body rise up as you push to arm lockout
13. Push your body directly backward toward the anchor
14. Use a purposefully slowed rep speed; "barely slowed"
15. Do not begin the push with a fast or explosive start
16. Use a continual "grind" rep speed; stay disciplined
17. Do not allow the elbows to flare while fighting through sticking points
18. Contract the triceps hard at every lockout

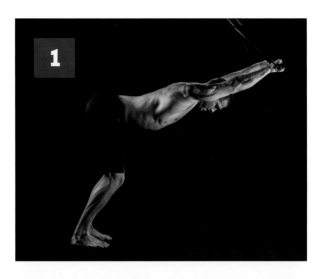

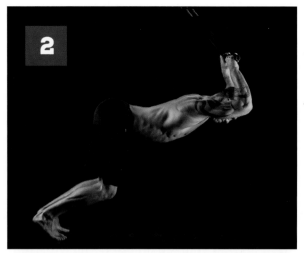

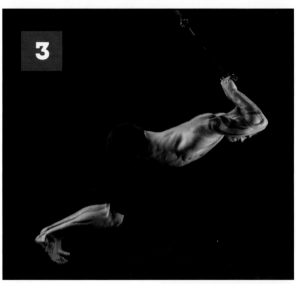

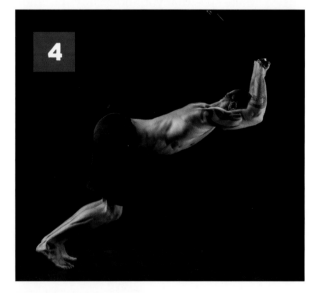

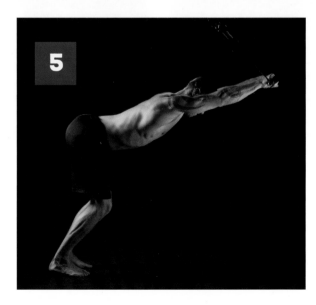

ONE-ARM ALTERNATING TRICEPS PRESS

The one-arm triceps press is light-years beyond the entry-level, two-arm triceps press in terms of difficulty. When the CrossCore® user shifts from the super stable two-arm triceps press (pin-in) to pulled-pin mode, the degree of difficulty exponentially increases. Shifting from two-arm to one-arm is dramatically more difficult: please use significantly less resistance. Setting your feet further away from the CrossCore® anchor-point while learning the one-arm triceps press will reduce the resistance and allow for the proper "ingraining" of perfect technique. We need precision without straining in order to learn this intricate exercise. Once the technique is mastered, resistance can be increased quickly.

1. The starting position is identical to the start of the two-arm triceps press
2. Lower yourself precisely and with tremendous control, using one-arm
3. Make sure that your body stays parallel to the floor
4. Relax at the bottom of the movement; feel the tri stretch
5. Push to a full and complete lockout using grind rep speed
6. Contract the triceps hard at lockout
7. "Rep out" on one-arm before switching arms
8. Avoid shortening the rep stroke as a shortened ROM yields stunted results
9. The trainee should "feel" the triceps work on descent and ascent

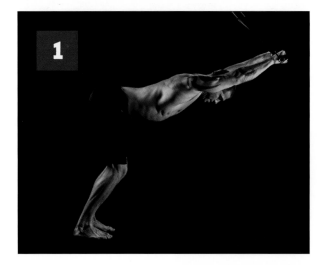
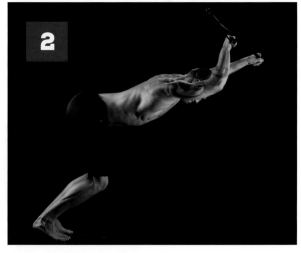

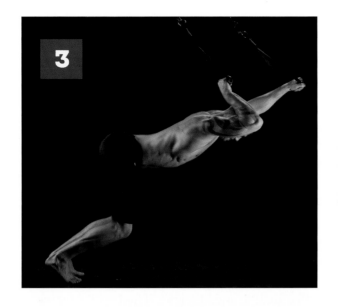

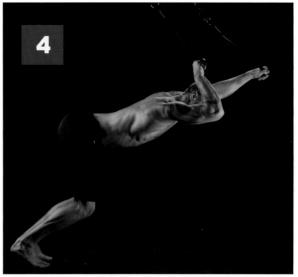

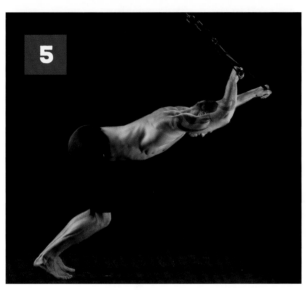

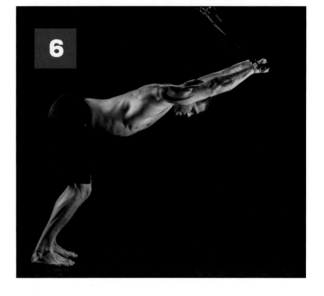

I-Y-T- REVERSE-Y PROGRESSIONS

This series of exercises derives from the traditional YTWL exercises taught by physiotherapists for shoulder rehabilitation. We have appropriated and modified the sequence for effective strength training with the CrossCore®.

Traditionally, these movements are performed while lying face down on a bench for support. Frequently the lower back can become hyperextended while performing these exercises on a bench. This can unnecessarily stress the lower back.

The CrossCore® HardCore I-Y-T-reverse Y progressions are performed upright in a rigid plank position (internal stabilization) with a neutral spine. This spares the back from hyperextension-related injuries. These progressions are excellent for building useful strength while stabilizing the scapulae (shoulder blades). Stable scapulae are essential for pain-free shoulder movement in sports and daily life. This sequence of exercises is both effective and efficient. The I-Y-T-reverse Y sequence corrects the "Upper Crossed Syndrome" discussed in the row progression.

These exercises are performed as a sequence. The "I" and "Y" require primary activation of the lower trapezius. The rhomboids and middle trapezius are activated in the "T" portion of the sequence. The "reverse Y" is a bilateral shoulder extension exercise that works several muscles including the latissimus dorsi, triceps, posterior deltoids, teres major and pectoralis major.

THE TWO-ARM I-Y-T- REVERSE-Y SEQUENCE:

1. Face the CrossCore® and lay back in planked position
2. Hands are held together, low and in front, knuckles face upward
3. For "I", slowly raise your arms overhead with only a slight bend at the elbows
4. At the final position hands are together overhead, shoulders are next to ears
5. Fight the negative as you lower arms back to starting position
6. Perform the prescribed number of reps for the "I"
7. "Y" raises both arms upward in a 45-degree angle
8. At the top of the movement the arms replicate the letter Y
9. Lower with tension, fight the negative
10. Perform the prescribed reps for the "Y" movement
11. "T" moves arms parallel to the ground as you pull
12. Knuckles should face behind you at the end of the T movement
13. Lower with tension; fight the negative
14. Perform the prescribed number of reps for the "T"
15. "Reverse Y" moves downward with palms facing behind
16. Perform the prescribed reps of the "reverse Y"
17. Perform an equal number of reps in each movement
18. Each movement needs to be crisp, consistent, and distinct

I SEQUENCE:

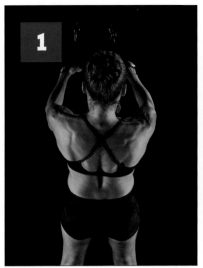
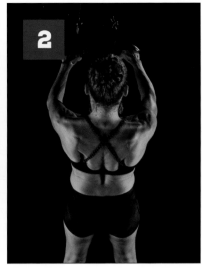
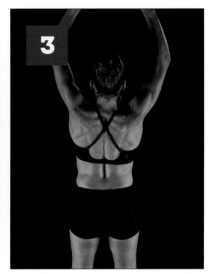

Y SEQUENCE:

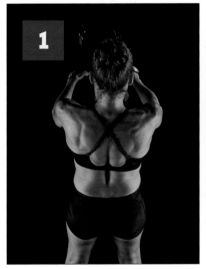
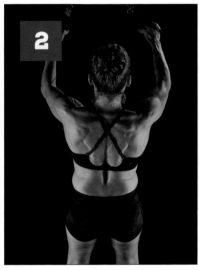
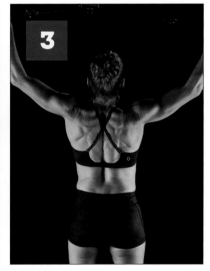

T SEQUENCE:

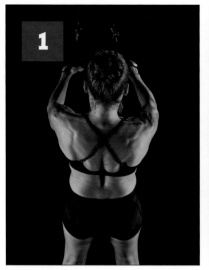
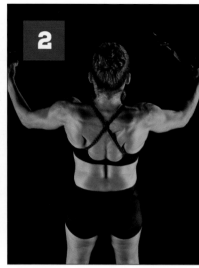
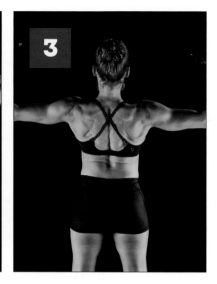

REVERSE Y SEQUENCE:

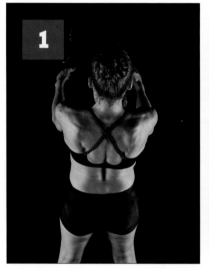
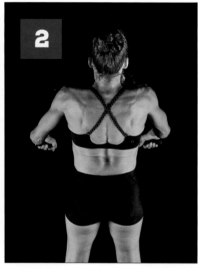
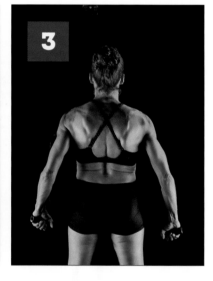

THE ONE-ARM I-Y-T- REVERSE-Y SPLIT VARIATION:

How do we make a difficult exercise more difficult? One method is to complete the same movement with only one hand at a time. This trick alone amps up the resistance to a dramatic degree; the trick is to maintain the same technique. Too often when switching from one to two arms, the CrossCore® user's technique breaks down. Be on guard against this. In the I-Y-T-Y sequence, the "split" procedure is to perform the target number of reps with one arm then immediately perform the identical movement with the other arm. For this exercise sequence, the specific procedure would be "I" movement, weak arm, strong arm; "Y" movement, weak arm, strong arm; "T" movement, weak arm, strong arm; "Reverse Y" movement, weak arm, strong arm.

1. Begin with the body in a plank position; arms in front, parallel to the ground
2. Start each movement phase with extreme contraction
3. Raise the weaker arm using grind speed
4. Keep the other arm straight out in front
5. Actively pull the shoulder back into the socket for stability
6. Control the eccentric (negative) phase of the movement
7. Switch hands and complete assigned reps
8. Complete the entire I-Y-T-r-Y sequence in this manner

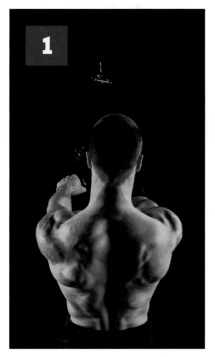 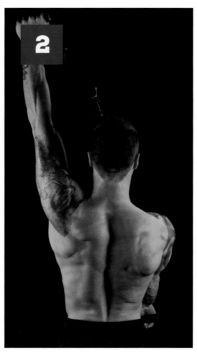 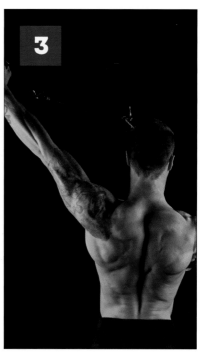

Starting position with end position of each movement

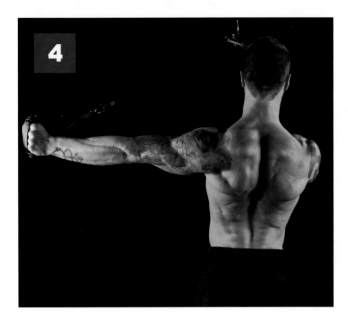
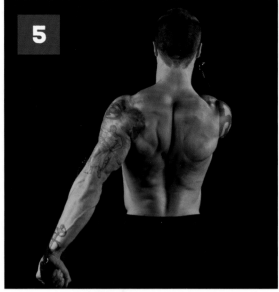

The one-arm split version of this exercise increases the degree of difficulty to a dramatic degree:

- Watch carefully for fraying or disintegrating technique
- Feel free to increase (or decrease) the resistance during or between reps
- Increases and decreases are easily made by moving the feet slightly
- No partial reps, rebounding, or using momentum. Grind each rep!
- Fight the negative—the resisted negative is as important as the concentric

SQUAT PROGRESSIONS

There are five distinctly different squat exercises in the CrossCore® HardCore program

1. Ultra-deep, two-leg squat with fixed pin or pulled pin
2. Airborne squat with pulled pin
3. Pistol squat with pulled pin
4. Dragon squat with pulled pin
5. Compound squat: airborne into pistol

DEVELOPING SQUATTING TECHNIQUE WITH CROSSCORE®

A good case could be made that the CrossCore® is the finest tool available anywhere for learning how to squat properly. Due to its unique ability to "lighten" a trainee's torso/payload, people who are new to squatting or who are otherwise unable to achieve a full range-of-motion while squatting are suddenly able to perform perfect, deep squats. Going deep is the secret to squat success. The deeper we go, the more muscle fiber we are able to stimulate. Full range-of-motion squatting creates leg and hip strength, the foundation of function and the requisite ingredient for athletic prowess.

If an athlete leans back against the CrossCore® handles as he or she descends in the squat, the weight of the torso can be significantly decreased. One wonderful phenomenon we have discovered is that obese, overweight, and weak individuals can use the CrossCore® to achieve wonderful, deep, full ROM squats in their very first session. A 200-pound individual carrying 40% body fat is usually unable to perform even a single full ROM body weight squat.

Using the CrossCore®, the out-of-shape are able to tug upwards on the handles as they encounter any squat sticking points. The unfit can literally pull their bodyweight through while maintaining perfect squat technique. The overweight and out of shape can effectively self-administer their own forced reps. An obese individual who is normally unable to perform a single deep squat is suddenly able to perform five to ten ultra-deep squat reps. Consistent CrossCore® squatting causes leg strength to skyrocket. We routinely see obese clients *double* their leg strength inside of four weeks.

ULTRA DEEP TWO-LEG SQUAT WITH FIXED PIN OR PULLED PIN

The finest single progressive resistance exercise is the squat, the deep knee bend, and all its mighty variants. Learn carefully these basic squat techniques, as all other squat variations are built atop these core squat techniques.

1.   Face the CrossCore® anchor point with knuckles facing upward
2.   Start with a shoulder width stance; do not make the stance too wide or narrow
3.   Use the CrossCore® to help maintain balance
4.   Break/bend at the knees: sit *back* and down—sitting back is critical
5.   Keep the knees pushed outward during both descent and ascent
6.   Optimally, the torso remains as vertical as possible
7.   Optimally the shins remain as vertical as possible
8.   Do NOT let the knees drift forward in front of the toes
9.   Inhale while sitting back and down in a controlled fashion
10.   When your thighs are parallel to the floor, exhale and sink further
11.   In the lowest position, the knees should be spread as wide as possible
12.   In the lowest position, the shins and torso should be as upright as possible
13.   Inhale and begin to stand erect—do not explode or jolt—power erect!
14.   Do not let the tailbone shoot up behind the torso to make rising easier
15.   With a vertical torso and knees pinned out, only the femurs move
16.   Power yourself erect using only the thighs and glutes
17.   Tug on the handles to provide as much "help" as needed
18.   Exhale during the concentric push phase
19.   Squat to a full lockout, making sure to flex your glutes
20.   Master fixed-pin squats before proceeding to pulled-pin squats

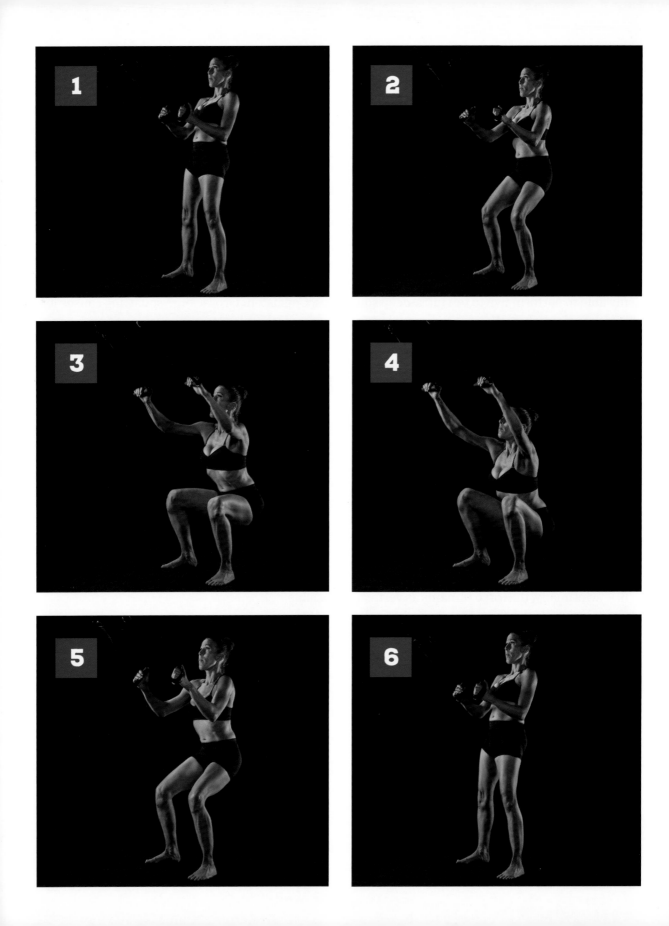

AIRBORNE SQUAT

For athletes in need of greater resistance than provided by regular CrossCore® squats, the airborne squat is the first of several difficult single-leg squat variants. These variants are designed to increase the resistance needed to complete a squat. In many cases, the single leg squat resistance can rival the muscular inroad created by barbell squatting. In many ways the airborne squat is technically the easiest single-leg squat to master, so we begin with it. The basic technique is to squat down on one thigh while extending the non-working foot behind you. Balance is key and stability will be built over time with practice. Use the CrossCore®handles to aid balance. The depth of the squat is limited by the rear leg, which makes the airborne squat the ideal entry-level single-leg squat.

1. Begin the airborne squat as you would a classic two-leg squat
2. Bend the knee of the working leg to begin the squat—sit back and down!
3. As the planted leg bends and lowers, the "free leg" is pushed behind the body
4. Use the CrossCore® handles as needed to maintain stability
5. Lower yourself on the working, planted leg with great control
6. The depth of the airborne squat is determined by the rear leg
7. Inhale in synchronization with the descent
8. The rear, non-working knee touches down behind the heel of the working leg
9. At the turnaround of the movement, push upward
10. Exhale as you arise
11. Do not allow your weight to shift forward over your toes on the working leg
12. "Rep out" on one leg before switching your stance
13. This initially awkward move will improve with practice
14. Make the rear leg knee touches light and precise

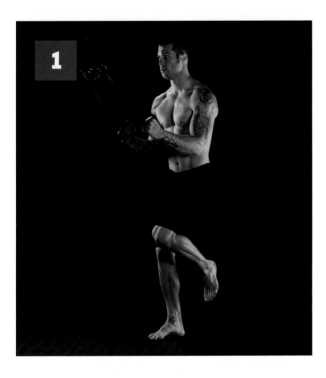
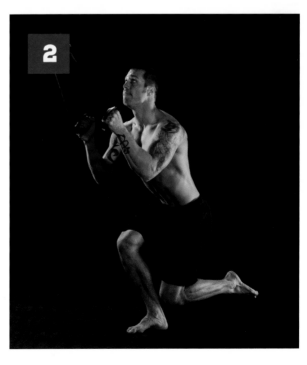

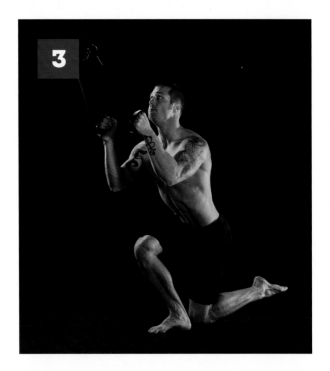

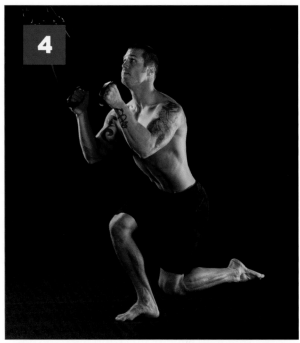

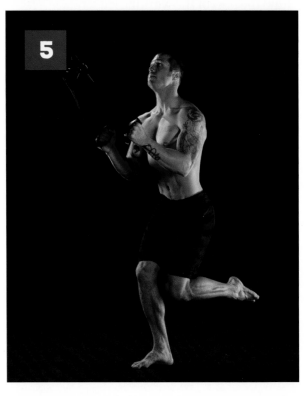

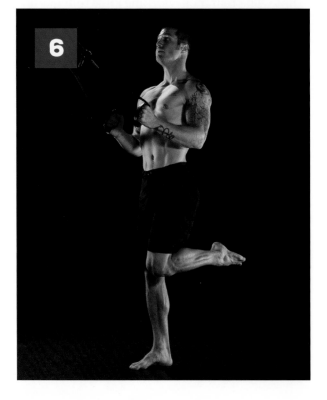

AIRBORNE SQUAT:
THE CURE FOR GLUTEAL AMNESIA

World-renowned biomechanics expert Dr. Stuart McGill coined the phrase, "gluteal amnesia" to describe an inability to activate the gluteal muscles during athletic and everyday movement. From a neuromuscular perspective, "forgetting" how to fire the gluteal muscles is a precursor to back, hip and knee injuries.

Gluteal amnesia sounds like a joke, but this phenomenon is epidemic—even amongst elite soldiers and world-class athletes. The sure-fire cure for those afflicted with gluteal amnesia is performing perfect airborne squats on a consistent basis.

The airborne squat is designed to maximize activation of the gluteal muscles in all movement planes. Most full-depth, two-leg squatting movements train the gluteus maximus primarily in one movement plane, hip extension. The airborne squat is a single-leg squat variant that needs to be performed with a very specific technique. When we bring the non-standing leg's knee down behind the heel of the working leg in the Airborne Squat, we are doing so for a reason—we want to recruit the maximum number of glute muscle fibers and keep them firing through multiple planes of movement.

As the non-standing leg moves behind the working leg, i.e., lowering into the squat, the working leg and hip move into internal rotation, adduction and flexion in relation to the pelvis. These three movements are the exact opposite of what the gluteus maximus does biomechanically—the gluteus maximus externally rotates, abducts, and extends the hip.

As we move downward during an airborne squat, the glutes of the working leg must eccentrically control the hip to prevent it from moving into extreme internal rotation, adduction, and flexion. This eccentric contraction triggers a tremendous activation of all the gluteus maximus muscle fibers and also strongly recruits the gluteus medius and minimus in their abduction (resisting adduction) function.

As we stand up from the lowest position of an airborne squat, the gluteal muscles of the working leg must fire and the effort is so intense every available glute fiber is needed to activate each tri-planar function.

As the athlete rises, they move out of an internally rotated, adducted and flexed hip position. The gluteal muscles are forced to fully activate to bring the hip back into a neutral position with the pelvis; this is done by externally rotating, abducting and extending the hip as the athlete stands.

This unique movement pattern, combined with a maximal range-of-motion, creates an intense neuromuscular stimulus that deeply affects the musculature. The airborne squat stabilizes the hip joint and builds incredible strength and torque.

Training the glutes with the airborne squat gives us a superior exercise that carries over into injury prevention and dramatically improves athletic performance. When the single-leg airborne squat is performed precisely and properly, we can stabilize and strengthen the hip in three different movement planes.

PISTOL SQUAT

The pistol is the classic single-leg squat. The CrossCore® makes the difficult pistol far easier by providing balance and stability. This stability enables the athlete to concentrate on squat *depth*. We will go all the way down on one leg using this squat variant. The CrossCore® HardCore techniques will enable the trainee to self-administer forced reps. By using the CrossCore®, people that are incapable of performing a single, unsupported pistol squat will now be able to perform multiple reps of assisted pistols for multiple sets. Over time, less and less "help" will be needed to arise. Each pistol repetition begins by squatting down as far as possible. Be sure to maintain proper technique throughout the movement since flawed technique will become ingrained if regularly repeated.

1. In the classic pistol squat, the non-standing leg is thrust forward
2. The heel of the non-standing foot does not touch the ground—or touches lightly
3. Use the handles of the CrossCore® to guide when sinking down
4. At the turnaround, pull on the handles to lighten the weight of your torso
5. Do not pull too much or too little when standing erect
6. The perfect pistol rep uses an even rep pace for concentric and eccentric

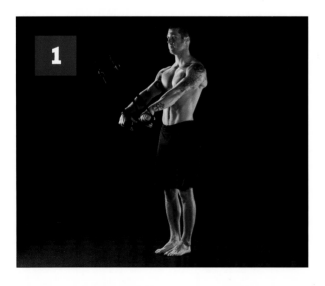
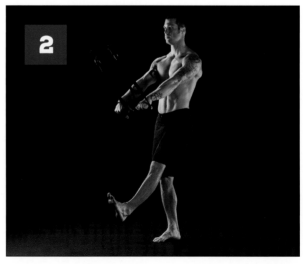

7. Inhale while descending and exhale while ascending
8. Make sure to complete a full lockout on every rep
9. Balance, position and rep pacing are critical to perform perfect pistols
10. Strive to continually master this difficult yet beneficial exercise

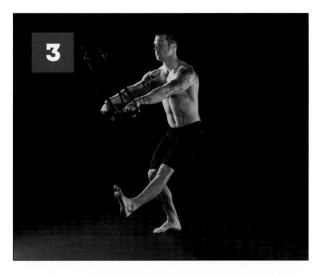
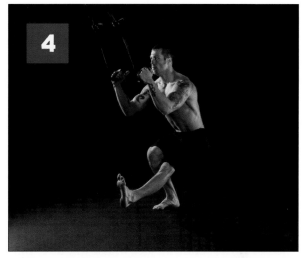
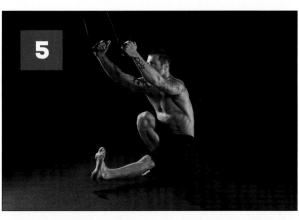
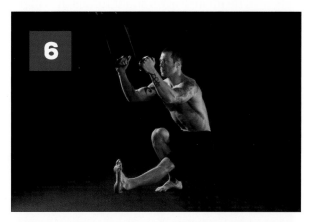
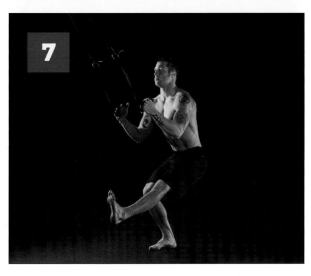
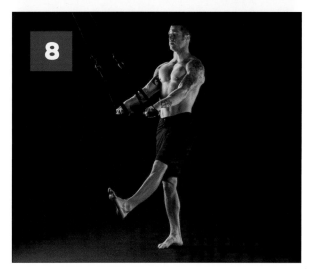

DRAGON SQUAT

This squat variant requires that the athlete rotate their entire torso and lightly touch the ground with the knee of the non-standing leg to conclude each rep. Squat depth is limited by the controlled knee touch, as seen in the photos. The dragon squat involves synchronizing the descent with a dramatic twist. The degree of difficulty is intense and needs to be experienced to gain a full understanding and appreciation of the movement. The dragon squat is an intentionally tough squat and if performed correctly, it is a valuable squat variant that should be practiced on a routine basis. Tracking, technique, position and control are the keys to perfecting dragon squats.

1. Have a clear mental picture of the technique used in the dragon squat
2. Clarity is critical for this most technically complex of all squats
3. Seek a smooth synchronization between the descending and twisting movements
4. Do not twist too much, do not twist too little
5. Lower yourself smoothly, powerfully and with control
6. Fight the tendency to want to free-fall and let gravity control the lowering
7. "Pull" yourself downward into the lowest position squat position
8. Do not contort, jerk or use undue explosiveness, use smooth power
9. The ideal dragon squat forces the thighs and glutes to power the movement
10. Be patient and precise; this technique is tricky but exceedingly productive
11. Rapid, sloppy twisting will create knee pain. Instead, move with deliberation
12. Make sure the twist leaves the torso facing sideways

The dragon squat's roots in martial arts are apparent. Many of the movements in the CrossCore® HardCore arsenal will have substantial benefit to the martial artist.

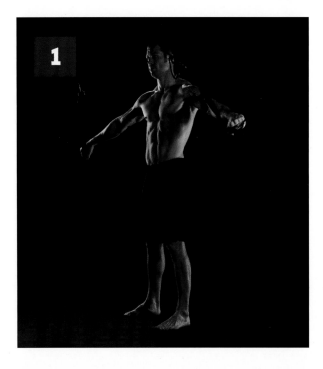
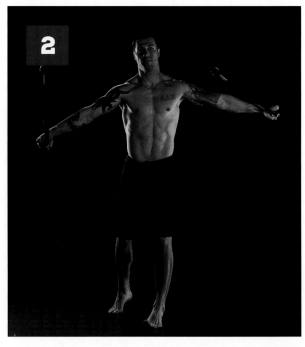

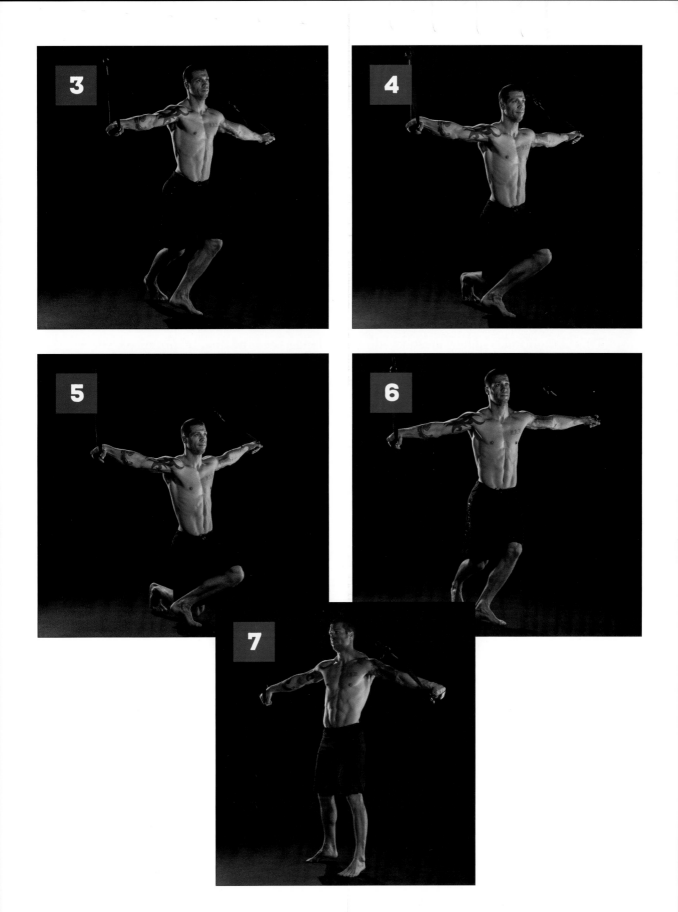

ABSOLUTE STRENGTH AND THE MARTIAL ARTIST

The physical requirements of a martial artist include flexibility, mobility, agility, speed, awareness, control and strength. Regardless the martial art, be it striking biased, grappling based or a weapon system—there is a need for strength in multiple capacities.

Unfortunately, most martial artists spend the majority of their training time practicing their art, doing aerobics, or working on their sustained strength, aka, strength endurance. When a martial artist is quizzed about lack of any "absolute strength" training, the stock answer is, "That's not the type of strength we want—we need sustained strength, strength endurance—the kind of strength that can be called upon late in a fight."

This contention is lunacy masquerading as science: the fundamental premise is flawed, yet no one points out the obvious. Absolute strength and sustained strength are not an either or proposition—as if the acquisition of one precluded attainment of the other.

Factually, absolute strength and sustained strength are two sides of the same strength coin. We want both. We can have both. Those that purposefully avoid absolute strength training do so at their own peril: this bias creates a chink in the armor, an Achilles heel, a literal weakness to be exploited by similarly skilled fighters that practice and possess absolute strength—in addition to copious amounts of complimentary sustained strength.

IF ABSOLUTE STRENGTH IS SUPERFLUOUS, WHY DO WE HAVE WEIGHT CLASSES?

Let us first explain the fallacy of the either/or strength premise that a sizeable percentage of contemporary martial artists subscribe to. It goes as follows, "I understand the need for strength but I don't need 500-pound bench press strength, I need lumberjack sustained strength. Ergo, 100% of my training time that I have apportioned to "strength training" will be filled with sustained strength drills: we'll push the prowler and wave ropes, we'll sprint and lift kettlebells, we'll inject an intense muscular effort into aerobic formats."

As Church Lady would say, "Well isn't that *special*."

Most of the avoiders of hardcore resistance training are worried about having the truth exposed about how physically weak they are. If everyone is using barbells and dumbbells, and you are so weak you have to use the 35 pound plates, that fact, your physical weakness, is betrayed to anyone watching. Now this same man can run a marathon and sprint up the side of a mountain carrying a 100-pound heavy bag. That is fine, wonderful and admirable; but it doesn't change the fact that he is a weak bitch. Rather than attack the weakness, better to rationalize that the need for this type of power is superfluous and not needed...

Really?

Let us construct a hypothetical situation using Krishnamurti-like deductive logic to reverse engineer a mind breakthrough...let us suppose BJ Penn will fight Cain Valazquez. BJ stands 5-9 and weighs 170 pounds. Cain stands 6-1 and weighs a lean and conditioned 240. On paper, Cain is in big trouble....

Athletic attributes		
	BJ	**Cain**
Speed	*	
Agility	*	
Flexibility	*	
Pure endurance	*	
Strength endurance	*	
Skills	*	
Experience	*	

Wow! This thing is so lopsided in BJ's favor that perhaps we should cancel this imaginary fight so BJ won't maim Cain. Oh, that is right—we forgot one single category...

Athletic attributes		
	BJ	**Cain**
Size and strength		*

And because of Cain's overwhelming superiority in one category, any fight between these two would be manslaughter: Cain would destroy BJ by simply holding him with one hand while pummeling him with a fist on the other hand like a concrete pumpkin. Cain would manhandle that far superior fighter, like a father enfolding a sixty-pound five-year old.

Let us put a finer point on the need for absolute strength: were BJ to fight an untrained 270-pound "normal person," BJ would destroy the civilian inside 60 seconds—factually we could eliminate "Size" out of "Size and strength."

The lone reason for Cain's easy dominance over a superior opponent is the massive imbalance in raw human power and strength.

Further, the acquisition of absolute strength, unlike other athletic attributes, can be dramatically increased with a minimum time investment. Two to three 20-minute sessions per week will in most cases, *double* the athlete's raw power and in a two to three month timeframe.

One final piece to the puzzle is the emergence of the CrossCore® as an effective and results-producing resistance training device. Now we can replicate the degree of muscular inroad produced by barbell/dumbbell free weight training using this unique portable device.

Our thought is, devoid the stigma of handling black iron, perhaps the CrossCore® can seduce martial artists into including and apportioning some training time (not much!) towards the pursuit of pure strength. The cutting-edge martial artist can use the CrossCore® to provide barbell/dumbbell workouts without the barbell/dumbbells. Now we can stop avoiding and denying that obvious chink in the martial armor and start addressing weaknesses instead of continually playing to our strengths.

Let us seek to build pure power using the CrossCore® in combination with our Old School HardCore protocols. Let us strive to rectify the gaping holes, the potentially disastrous gaps, all due to the crime of negligence.

The CrossCore® will be a game changer within the martial arts world. For the first time, martial artists have access to a tool that allows them to move and generate force from a multitude of positions and angles—just like in a real conflict. Developing both unilateral and bilateral strength in multiple planes using variable load, will enable the athlete to fill in the blanks in their martial skill set. We need it—and with a minimum time investment.

COMPOUND SQUAT

Our final squat variation combines the deep and difficult pistol squat with the less difficult, but still demanding airborne squat. First, perform a pistol squat then, still standing on the same leg, immediately perform the airborne squat. One pistol + one airborne squat = one rep. This unique combination stimulates the muscles of the thighs and glutes in a way that will tax even the strongest conventional barbell squatter. We have had men capable of raw squatting 600 pounds with a barbell fail when performing a set of single-leg compound squats. This should give you an idea of how difficult this variation is, and the degree of muscular tension generated by this 1-2 punch compound squat.

Immediately end the set if technique breaks down. The dividing line between results and injury is a razor's edge. Empirical experience has repeatedly shown that most progressive resistance injuries occur when a fatigued lifter insists on continuing to perform reps after their technique has disintegrated.

1. Compound squats are the last word in CrossCore® squat difficulty
2. Maintain perfect technique as you perform the pistol
3. Maintain perfect technique as you morph into the airborne squat
4. When performing compound squats, avoid rushing through them
5. Each of the two component squats need to be precise
6. Adhere to all the technical parameters associated with both squat variations
7. Descend and perform a perfect pistol squat, exhale as you rise
8. At the top of the pistol, inhale and begin the airborne squat
9. Touch the unloaded knee lightly behind the foot of the standing leg
10. Exhale as you stand back up from the airborne squat
11. The non-stop combination of pistol and airborne squat completes ONE rep
12. It is better to perform one rep with perfect form than five sloppy reps
13. Each squat variation need be mastered separately and sequentially
14. Don't jump ahead and start doing compound squats before you are ready
15. This intense combination works thighs, glutes and even hamstrings
16. Develop a smooth flow as you crank out reps of compound squats

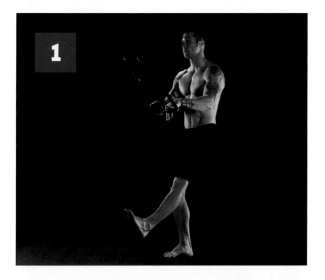
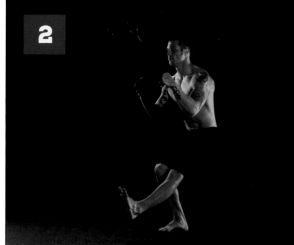
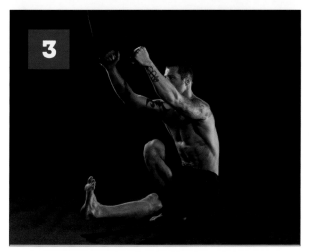
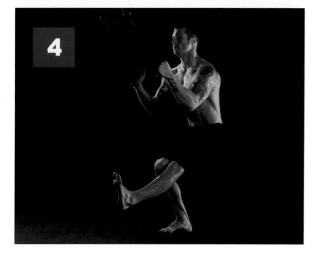

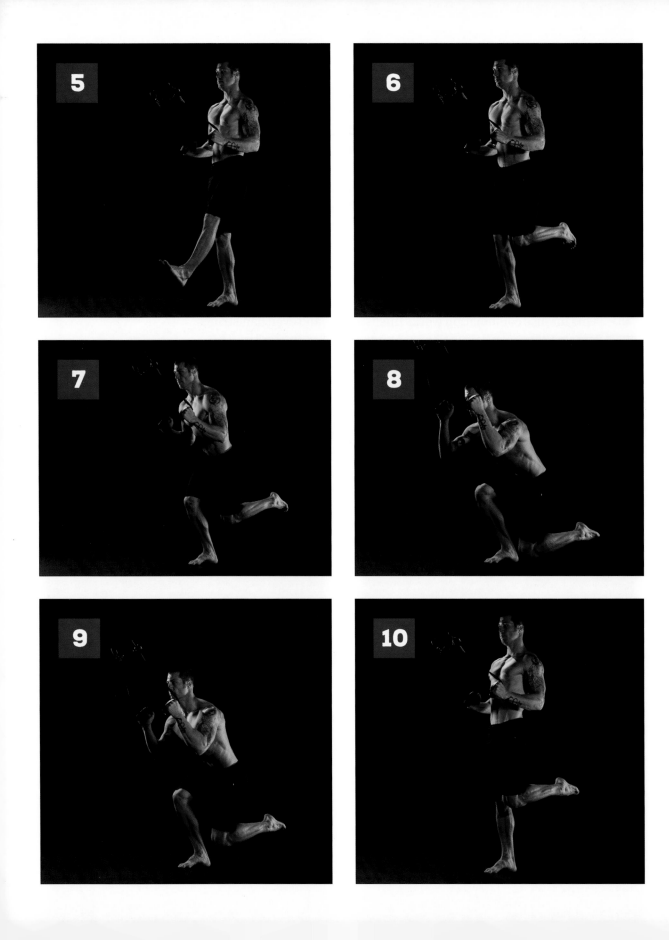

EXERCISE TECHNIQUES

VERTICAL ANCHOR EXERCISES

DEAD BUG ROW

This is a gymnastic or acrobatic movement where the trainee rows while suspended upside down. Obviously this is an advanced move that forces the rower to use 100% of their bodyweight while rowing. Take great care to make sure you are doing this movement correctly, or it will be completely ineffective.

THIS IS A VERY ADVANCED EXERCISE *and should only be attempted by a seasoned CrossCore® HardCore veteran. The beginner trainee has no business performing this exercise. The abdominal strength, body control and rowing strength necessary for the safe performance of this movement must be developed through months (or years) of consistent training.*

1. Place padding below you, especially if working over hard flooring
2. Shorten the rope so that your inverted torso will clear the ground
3. Grab the handles and curl your legs inward and upward
4. You should now be in a ball
5. Shoulders are rounded with your legs and feet tucked in tight
6. Row with one arm to lift your entire body toward the ceiling
7. Make sure to feel the lats contracting as you pull
8. Pull as high as possible, lower yourself back down with precision and care
9. Repeat the movement with the other arm
10. Achieve a balance point so that only your lats are powering the lift
11. In order for the lats to fire, the rep stroke needs to be more than a few inches

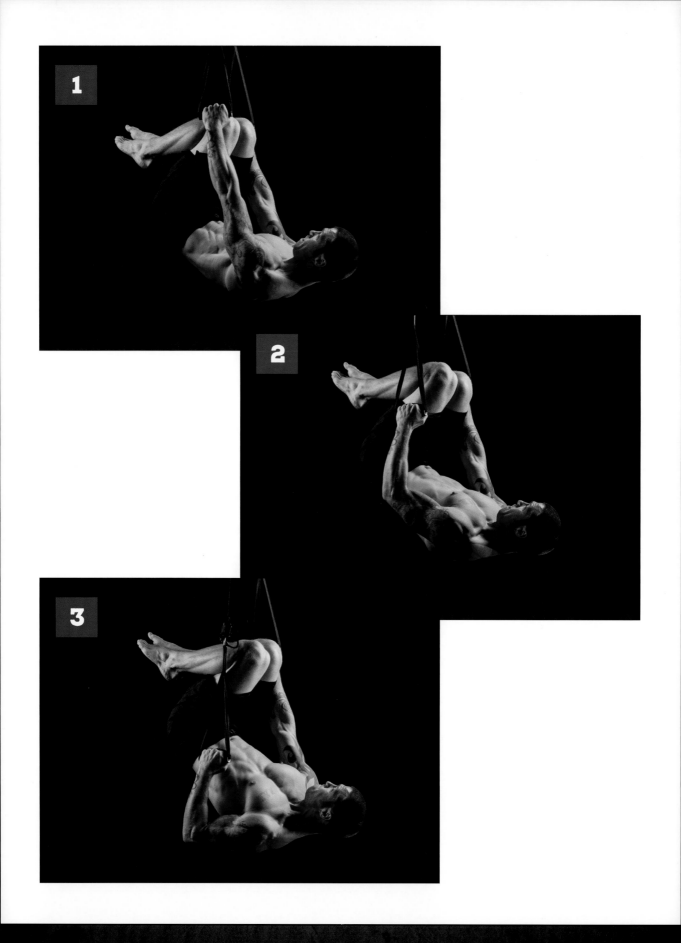

DIP PROGRESSIONS

The mighty dip with all its varieties and types has been a staple of progressive resistance training since the 1950s. Back then, power-bodybuilders like Marvin Eder (who once performed a single dip with 440 pounds attached to his waist), Reg Park and Bill Pearl popularized the "weighted dip." Hardcore powerlifters like Pat Casey, the first man to bench press 600 pounds, used heavy dipping to increase their triceps power and to build lower pec power. The dip—performed correctly—needs to be "deep" enough to stimulate and engage the triceps. If it is too shallow the dip is rendered ineffective. The classic dip descends to a point where, when viewed from the side, the upper arm is slightly below parallel to the floor. The body is pushed upward to a full and complete lockout. Ultra-deep dipping, a more advanced technique, requires lower pectoral engagement to "power out" of the lowest position and push upward to the point where the triceps take over.

SEATED DIP

Not everyone is capable of doing dips. Heavy individuals are at the same disadvantage for dips as they are for chin-ups or pull-ups. Obviously a 200-pound individual must push a lot more dip weight than someone that only weighs 100 pounds. The CrossCore® allows everyone the opportunity to explore this incredible exercise whether or not they are able to do classic dips. The secret is to use the feet to reduce the weight of the dipper while dipping. The "seated dip" is an entry-level variation that is perfect for learning how to dip properly while simultaneously working towards the classic dip. In pulled-pin mode, the challenge of the seated dip is made greater because of the added instability.

1. The CrossCore® anchor point is directly overhead
2. Set up the strap length so the CrossCore® handles dangle at waist height
3. Grab the handles and keep them close to the body throughout the movement
4. The handles can be held facing front to back, or sideways
5. The classic dip is performed with the handles facing front-to-back
6. The "sideways" dip is performed with the knuckles facing forward
7. Each hand position is equally difficult
8. Each hand position has a slightly different muscular effect
9. Place the feet roughly one foot in front of the torso with knees bent
10. Bend at the elbows and lower down with great care
11. Do not let your arms stray outward, lower straight down
12. When the upper arms are roughly parallel to the floor, push back upward
13. Apply as much pressure with your feet as needed to complete the rep
14. Attain a full and complete "hard" lockout at the top of each and every dip rep
15. Inhale while lowering, exhale while pushing upward
16. Over time, use less downward leg pressure to complete each dip
17. Master fixed-pin mode before progressing to pulled-pin mode

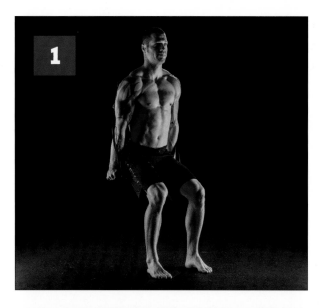

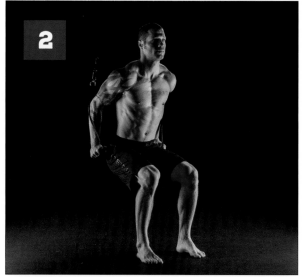

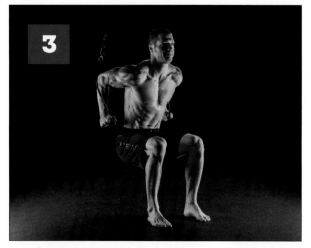

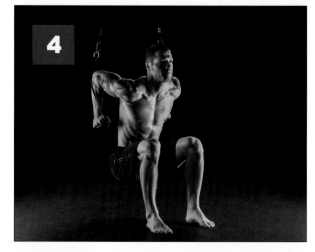

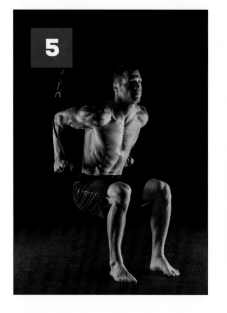

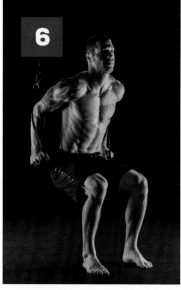

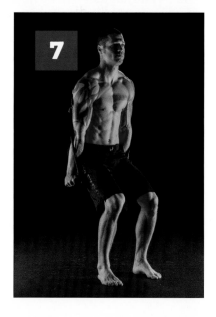

The seated dip can be made more difficult by gradually straightening the supporting legs. The most advanced position has no bend in the knees, with the legs straight out in front. Over time, the trainee no longer needs to bend the knees. Over time, the feet exert less and less downward pressure until, eventually, the dipper no longer need any self-assistance. They are now ready for the suspended dip.

SUSPENDED DIP

If the athlete becomes strong enough, they will eventually be able to dip while bearing the weight of the entire body. Dipping with the unstable handles of the CrossCore® is far more difficult than dipping between two *fixed* parallel bars. The inherent instability of the constantly moving, swaying dip handles makes the difference between a seated dip and a suspended dip a wide, wide chasm. One trick used by pros is to very lightly touch the floor with their toes while mastering suspended dips. This light touch prevents swaying and makes dipping much easier. But even while using this trick, CrossCore® dipping is extremely tough compared to fixed parallel bar dipping—especially in pulled-pin mode.

1. Observe all the preliminary rules outlined for seated dips
2. Pin-in please
3. Use the transitional technique: lightly touch the floor with your toes or heels
4. Dip down carefully until your arms are slightly below parallel
5. Push upward to a full and complete lockout
6. Over time, experiment with less and less foot or toe touch
7. Ultimately, dip with your feet totally off the floor
8. Master the fixed-pin mode before progressing to the pulled-pin mode

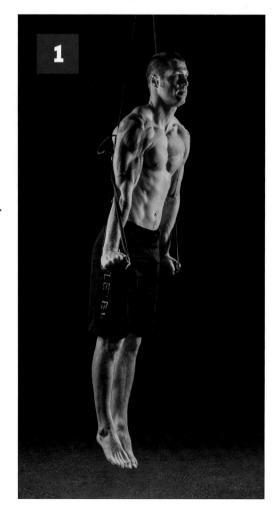

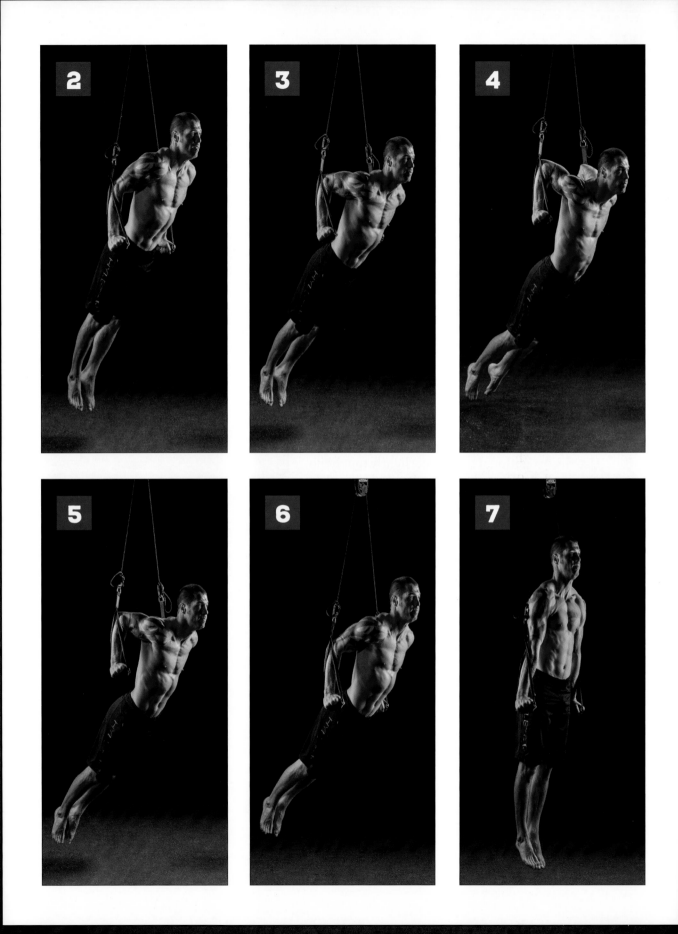

For the advanced trainee, there are many ways to further increase resistance with the dip.

1. Shift from the fixed-pin set up to pulled-pin for a much greater stability challenge
2. Slow down the rep speed—slower is harder
3. Dip deeper. Go as far down as humanly possible to activate the pecs
4. Wear a weighted vest for the ultimate in resistance

ABDOMINAL PROGRESSIONS

The biggest lie in all of fitness is that targeted abdominal exercises will melt away the body fat that lies atop the waistline. Prolonged abdominal exercise is erroneously credited with melting away the body fat that obscures the abdominal muscles. Hundreds of crunches or leg raises would—over a very long time—melt away gut fat to reveal six-pack abs. But, unfortunately for humanity, ripped abs are factually the result of attaining a low body fat percentage. Diet and nutrition, combined with intense exercise, is the avenue used by experts to lower body fat and thereby melt the obscuring body fat off the abs.

Still, we need to work our abdominal muscles, which need to be built and strengthened, just like any other muscles. We should not neglect them, but we should not overemphasize them. We also want to train the abdominals to strengthen their function as anterior core stabilizers. The CrossCore® HardCore abdominal progressions (especially the dynamic plank variations) are superb and appropriate for this purpose.

The CrossCore® is a superior ab training tool, able to attack the entire core from an unlimited number of angles and with great intensity and precision. To isolate any section of the ab core, it is crucial to find the correct angle and feel the targeted muscle working. We exploit proper pathways and once we find the perfect groove, imprint it. We will work our abs hard—but without any illusions.

KNEE RAISE

The knee raise will be challenging for most CrossCore® trainees at first; you will be contending with a wide array of forces, all of which will require the athlete to create stabilization in all planes. We will be forced to develop transitional skills that enable and allow smooth sequential execution of the various techniques. One of the key factors in executing the knee raise technique is to minimize the amount of swinging that can occur. The only way to do this is to keep absolute control over the beginning and ending positions. In the beginning position, the athlete needs to brace himself in the straps with his feet pointed slightly to the front. The body should be in this "hollow" position. This is also the ending position and must be returned to forcefully and consciously. This is done by driving the feet and legs forward.

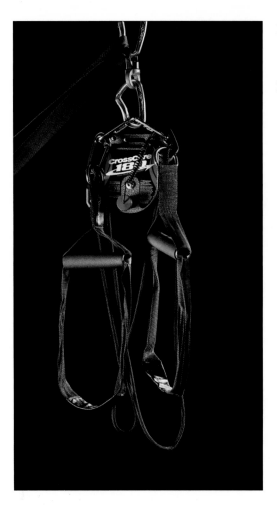

1. Attach the CrossCore® carabiners to the metal anchor loops on each side of the device (seen at left)

2. To begin the knee raise, extend the handle straps as far as possible (below)

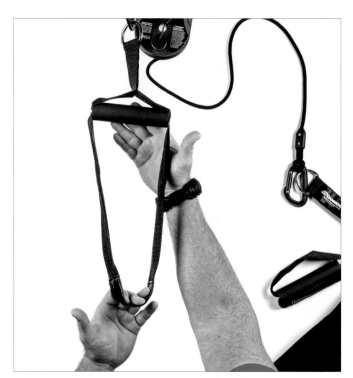

3. Put your arms through the new opening
4. Grasp the handles or ropes in a comfortable position
5. While the body is in an upright position, create tension in the abs
6. Stabilize the "hollow" position by pointing your feet slightly to the front
7. Maintain a strict upright position, slowly bring your knees up to the chest
8. Contract the abs hard
9. Support the torso with an equally forceful contraction of the glutes
10. Use a grind rep speed
11. Hold the contracted position at the top
12. Reverse the movement and return to the starting position
13. Grind on the way down: think of this as a continual tension exercise
14. Point the feet at a spot in front of the body to reduce swaying
15. From the starting position bring your knees to your chest

LEG RAISE

Once you are familiar with the knee raise and have mastered maintaining the "hollow" position needed to reduce swaying, you are now ready to move onto the leg raise. The leg raise is a significant step up in difficulty. The strength required to perform this movement smoothly will take time to develop. The leg raise is also called the "L-Sit" in gymnastics and is an indicator of extreme positional strength and control of midline and abs. Like the Knee Raise, particular attention must be used to control the transition in and out of the starting and ending positions. No momentum or "snap" should be used.

1. To begin the leg raise, extend the handle straps as far as possible
2. Insert your arms through the new opening
3. Grasp the handles or straps using a comfortable hand position
4. With the body in an upright position, create tension in the abs
5. Stabilize the "hollow" position
6. Feet are slightly in front and pointed towards the ground
7. Maintain a strict upright position, slowly raise the legs to a 90-degree angle
8. Movement is created by forcefully contracting the abs
9. Support the torso with an equally forceful contraction of the glutes
10. Perform the movement using grind rep speed
11. Hold the extended position
12. Reverse the movement and return to the starting position
13. Use grind rep speed on the way down
14. Point the feet at a spot in front of the body to reduce swaying

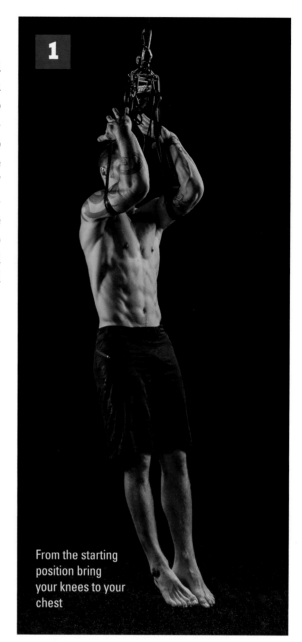

1

From the starting position bring your knees to your chest

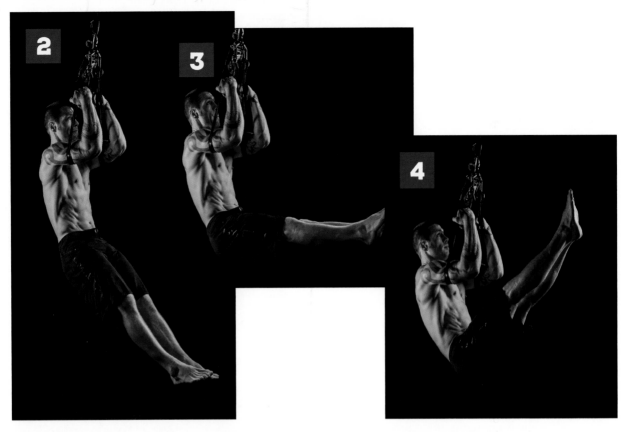

The leg raise can be made more difficult by extending the range of motion until you ultimately can point your feet at the ceiling.

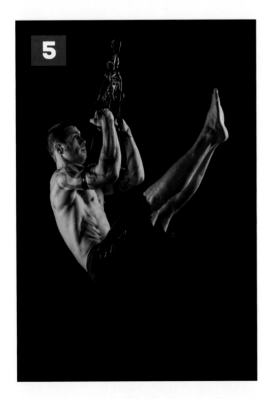

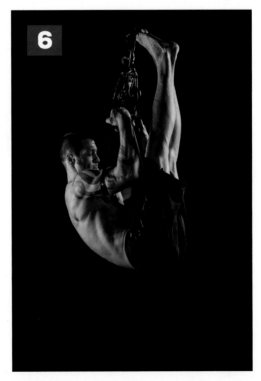

THE DYNAMIC PLANK

The dynamic plank requires the trainee stabilize and control each lower limb (in space) against the instability of the pulled-pin mode. The position of the legs must be maintained while bringing the entire lower body through multiple planes of movement while performing each exercise variation. A properly performed dynamic plank will maximally fire every prime mover and stabilizer of the core. Ten reps of this sequence while following the CrossCore® HardCore technique checklist will set the core on fire without the risk of injury to the back.

DYNAMIC PLANK (KNEE TUCK)

The first variation of the dynamic plank is the knee tuck. This is the easiest variation of the three and works the core with movement in the sagittal plane.

1. Set up the CrossCore® in the vertical anchor position
2. The straps on the handle hang at about knee height from the ground
3. Sit on the ground and place your feet in the straps
4. Flip around: you are lying in the prone position on your abdomen
5. The bottoms of your feet are against the handles
6. The tops of your feet are supported by the straps
7. You will need to experiment to attain perfect strap adjustment
8. Assume a plank position with your hands directly under your shoulders
9. Move forward or backwards in relation to the anchor
10. Heels are in a horizontal line with your upper back
11. The line formed from your upper back to your heels is parallel to the floor

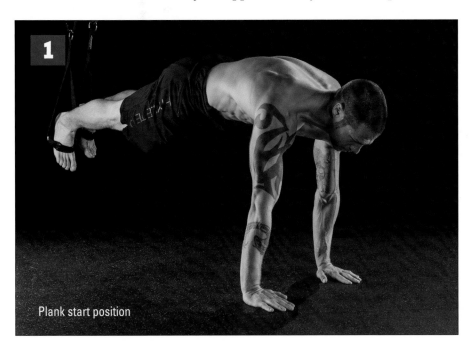

Plank start position

12. Perform the movement by bringing your knees to the back of your arms
13. Use grind speed
14. Briefly pause in the top position
15. Lower yourself back to the plank position
16. Return to the plank position
17. Do not let your back hyperextend as you return to the starting plank position
18. Technique MUST be maintained at all times
19. Repeat the movement for the designated number of reps

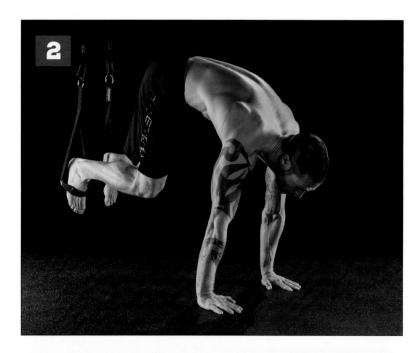

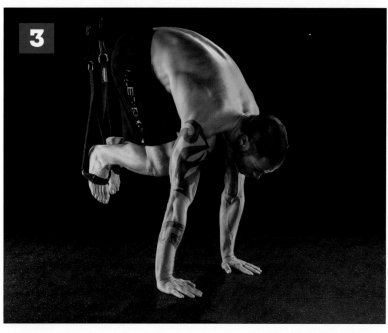

DYNAMIC PLANK (PIKE POSITION)

The level of difficulty is increased with the "pike" variant of the dynamic plank. The straight, locked legs create a mechanical disadvantage that must be overcome by generating more force from the abdominal muscles. This movement is also incredibly effective for improving shoulder strength and stability, since the finished position resembles a modified handstand.

1. The setup and start positions are identical to the knee tuck dynamic plank
2. Keep the legs locked at the knees
3. Start the movement by hinging at the hips
4. Pull your locked legs toward the back of your arms as one unit
5. The hips rise toward the ceiling at grind speed
6. The top position will look a lot like a modified handstand
7. Pause briefly then descend to the starting position at grind speed
8. Control the descent, avoid hyperextension of the spine (losing the plank)
9. Repeat for the predetermined amount of repetitions

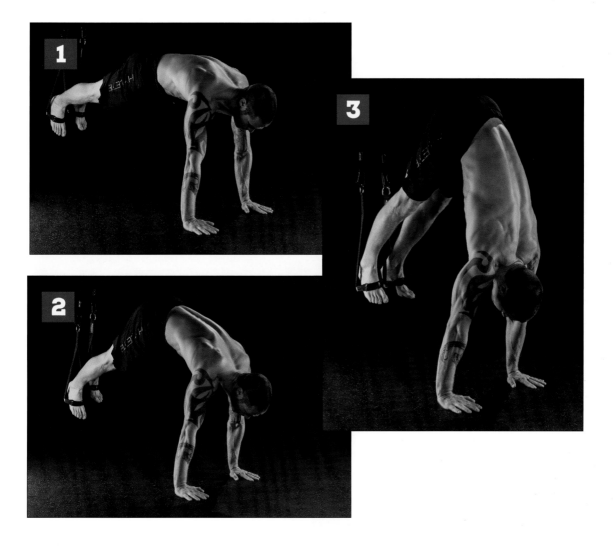

DYNAMIC PLANK (OBLIQUE)

The oblique variant of the dynamic plank adds movement in the transverse plane to an already difficult sagittal plane exercise. The amount of core control and strength needed to properly perform this variation makes this the most challenging and advanced of the three plan variants.

1. The setup and start position is identical to the knee tuck dynamic plank
2. From the start position, rotate the body below the waist as far as possible
3. The kneecaps are pointing to the left
4. Maintain the position of your upper body
5. Bring both of your knees as close as possible to the back of your left arm
6. Use grind speed
7. Pause in the top position briefly
8. Return to the starting position
9. Control the descent
10. Avoid back hyperextension at completion of the movement
11. Repeat the sequence now rotating to the right side
12. Alternate left and right side movements for the predetermined repetitions

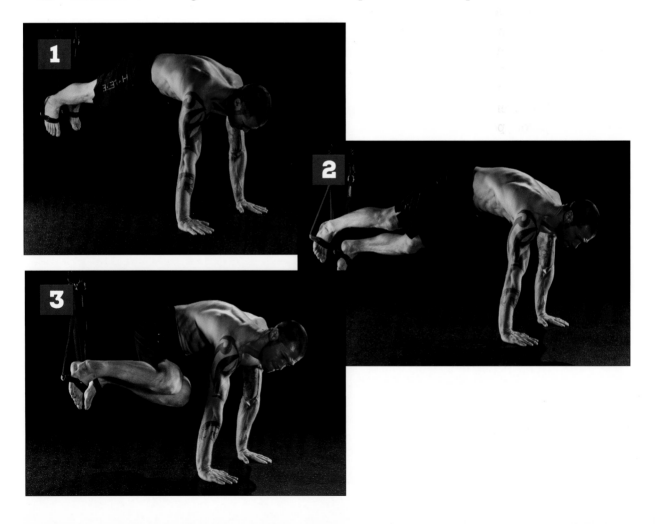

LEG CURLS

Leg curls with the CrossCore® will make the uninitiated feel as weak as a kitten and, at first, unable to do more than a few pristine reps. Persevere as strong, powerful hamstrings are critical for maximal speed when sprinting, height when jumping, distance when leaping or needed power when exploding upward in any athletic manner or fashion.

The CrossCore® offers the user a fantastic hamstrings exercise—assuming the athlete is able to master the technique. This is a tough one: you must lie on your back, slip your feet into the straps and play with the movement until you make the mind/muscle, or in this case the hamstring/brain connection.

This movement requires control of the abs and glutes to maintain the starting and ending positions. Start with the CrossCore® in fixed-pin mode and progress to pulled-pin after you have learned and mastered the movement. Pulled-pin mode will also allow for a single leg variation.

1. Extend the handle straps just far enough to insert your heels into the gaps
2. Allow your insteps to rest against the handles
3. Adjust the strap length as necessary to accommodate this position
4. Lie back and place your hands on the ground beside the body
5. Press down with your heels to raise the hips off the ground
6. The weight of your body is balanced between the heels and the shoulders
7. There should not be pressure on the neck or head in this position
8. If there is, then move closer to the CrossCore®
9. Change your point of focus to between the legs
10. The knees are extended with the heels pointing towards the ground
11. Forcefully drive the heels down and towards the buttocks
12. Allow the knees to bend and the hips to rise
13. Feel the hamstrings contract
14. Pull to completion
15. When the movement stops; reverse gears
16. Maintain grind rep speed throughout the movement
17. Return to the start by slowly pushing the heels away from the buttocks
18. Knees are back in an extended position

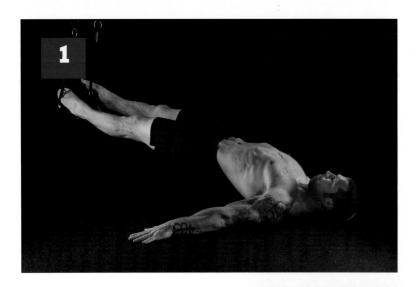

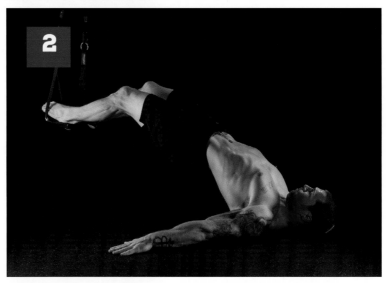

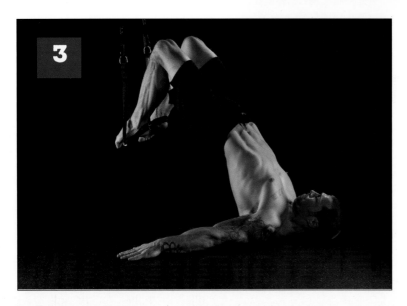

PART III

PLAN OF
ATTACK

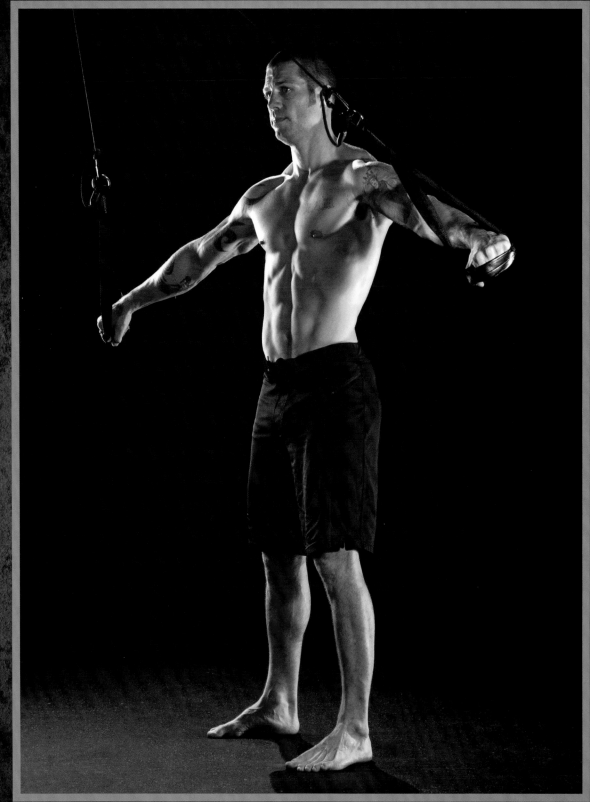

TACTICAL PLAN OF ATTACK

TOOLS AND TECHNIQUES WITHOUT TACTICS ARE WORTHLESS. WE NEED A PLAN.

There is a difference between "exercising" and "training." The general public exercise when they go to the health club or Y. They perform a few randomly selected progressive resistance movements, machines preferred; the average fitness devotee lifts distractedly, halfheartedly, exerting submaximal effort, often holding conversations while they are training or texting between sets. This is exercising.

Training is something an elite athlete does in order to increase power and strength and ergo, overall human performance. Training is preplanning: where are we at, physically? What are our current capacities? Where do we want to get to—realistically—how long until we get there? Once an elite athlete selects a realistic goal, they set the goal into a timeframe.

Each successive training week, more is expected of the athlete in their progressive resistance sessions. We need be realistic and egoless when we establish goals. Generally, tactically, philosophically speaking, we start off below capacity, develop techniques and create momentum. We end the specified time period 2-10% above previous capacities. Often the end of these strength cycles coincides with a competition, tryout or event.

Training requires preplanning; we construct a template set within a timeline and adhere to it. Experience has shown that intense desire for physical change generates motivation; this motivation is the spark that lights the tinder that starts the transformative fire. Once the burning desire, the motivation for dramatic physical change takes root, we execute the battle plan with the needed tenacity, perseverance and methodic application—this is not a battle this is a siege—we need attain and maintain a continuous effort lasting 6-16 weeks with an average elite strength peaking/muscle-building *training* cycle being 12 weeks in length.

Periodization, programming, is synonymous with preplanning. Programming for our purposes is a cohesive strength strategy for systematically building and strengthening muscle. A proper, periodized training regimen is called a "cycle" and is a roadmap, a game plan for dramatic physical transformation.

A periodized game plan consists of parallel and synchronized elements that run, unfold and progress, simultaneous and synchronized with each other. Our goal is to impart the knowledge as to how to create effective progressive resistance training protocols for the CrossCore®.

What good is a resistance-training workout if the degree of effort is halfhearted and insufficient to invoke the adaptive response? If hypertrophy is not triggered, if no strength gains are acquired, no muscle built, then why are we working out? We might as well be golfing or bowling. Training requires ever increasingly elevated degrees of effort: each succeeding week you exert harder and the harder you exert the greater the adaptive response and ergo, the greater the tangible gains.

Periodization, programming, pre-planning for athletics, has its own unique language, slang and insider lingo. Programming establishes various categories; each category has some sort of benchmark that we seek to improve upon each successive week over the life of the cycle. Periodization requires preplanning and the ongoing logging and notating of results as the "process" proceeds.

Frequency	How many times per week do we train?
Duration	How long is the workout session?
Intensity	How hard do we work during the session?
Sets & reps	How many reps per set?
Rep speed	How fast or how slow are the reps performed?
ROM	How long or short is the rep stroke Range-Of-Motion?
Content	What specific exercises are performed during the session?
Techniques	What specific techniques are used and why?

So how does a classical periodized cycle look? For these purposes we have created a "four column" 12-week periodized cycle of four exercises: two barbell and two CrossCore® movements. In columns 1 and 3 we plot barbell bench pressing and barbell squatting and in columns 2 and 4, we cycle two CrossCore® exercises, the chest press and three types of single-leg squatting. Our hypothetical athlete commenced his cycle with a 175-pound maximum bench; he begins benching 15% under capacity and ends up a benching a full 17% above capacity. He begun his barbell squat cycle able to perform a 250 x 1 squat: he starts squatting 30% under capacity and ends up 20% above capacity with a 300 x 1 effort.

Bench press	CrossCore® chest press	Squat	CrossCore® squats
Week 1 150x8	one set 5 reps	175x8	pistol, two sets of 5
Week 2 155x8	one set 6 reps	185x8	pistol, two sets of 6
Week 3 160x8	one set 7 reps	195x8	pistol, two sets of 7
Week 4 165x8	one set 8 reps	205x8	pistol, two sets of 8
Week 5 170x5	two sets 7 reps	225x5	compound squat 2x6
Week 6 175x5	two sets 8 reps	235x5	compound squat 2x7
Week 7 180x5	two sets 9 reps	245x5	compound squat 2x8
Week 8 185x5	two sets 10 reps	255x5	compound squat 2x10
Week 9 190x4	three sets 9 reps	265x4	backpack pistol 2x5*
Week 10 195x3	three sets 10 reps	275x3	backpack pistol 2x5
Week 11 200x2	three sets 11 reps	285x2	backpack pistol 2x5
Week 12 205x1	three sets 12 reps	300x1	backpack pistol 2x5

During weeks 9 thru 12, the pistol squatter wears a backpack or weighted vest: each successive week the squatter adds 10 to 20 pounds to the backpack or increases the weight of the weighted vest.

Take note of the structure and flow. The wise athlete starts off light and well below capacity and ingrains the precise techniques required. We build momentum so that by the end of the 12-week periodized cycle, the athlete exceeds all previous best efforts. The body gradually acclimatizes to ever greater degrees of effort and workload; by sequentially and systematically handling these ever-increasing training demands, the body grows, strengthens and adapts.

CROSSCORE® BEGINNER, INTERMEDIATE AND ADVANCED TACTICS

BEGINNER:
TWICE OR THRICE WEEKLY CROSSCORE® 'WHOLE BODY WORKOUT'

As a beginner new to CrossCore®, we recommend that you use an identical workout template two or even three times per week. The workout is identical on purpose: we want the trainee to focus on a limited menu of key and critical CrossCore® exercises. Rather than do countless exercises haphazardly, we concentrate on doing fewer exercise but doing them 'better.' We strive to improve exercise technique session-to-session, week-to-week. We seek to improve our focus and we learn the art of 'psyching.'

Do not change the exercise order as these exercise are sequenced in this particular way for a reason. Minimally, we perform this workout twice a week. Optimally we hit this workout three times a week for four straight weeks. These are the most basic and important of all the CrossCore® exercises. By doing them two to three times a week, we drill technique hard and often and accelerate the learning curve dramatically and radically.

THE WORKOUT

- **Squat, two-leg**
- **Chest Press, two-arm**
- **Row, two-arm**
- **I-Y-T-rY**
- **Curl, two-arm**
- **Triceps extension, two-arm**
- **Dynamic plank (knee-tuck)**

WORKOUT FACTOIDS

The exercises used in the beginner template are the most basic and the most important of all CrossCore® HardCore exercises. These exercises and their variations, form the bedrock techniques for CrossCore® HardCore. Beginners should do this workout a minimum of twice weekly with three times per week being optimal. Twice-a-week training sessions are separated by three or four days of rest. Thrice weekly sessions can be done Monday/Wednesday/Friday or Tuesday/Thursday/Sunday. Three times per week is 33% better than twice weekly—more is better as more training accelerates the learning curve. We use a purposefully limited number of exercises. Two sets are done for each exercise. We perform a light 'warm-up' set followed (after resting) by a second, 'all out' set. The first set consists of easy reps done using a gentle angle, a full ROM and a grind rep speed. The second set is all out and each exercise ideally concludes with a barely completed final rep. This maximal intensity set is called the 'all out top set.' Seek to adhere to periodized goals and over time we push past present limits and capacities in every exercise session.

1. You may use either a "Straight Set" or "Giant Set" strategy
2. Straight sets: perform all the sets for an exercise, then move on
3. Giant sets: one exercise is followed by the different exercise, without pause
4. Straight sets do not "trump" giant sets—or vice versa—just tools in the toolbox
5. We purposefully *avoid* pausing in this particular beginner workout
6. Do not pause when concentric becomes eccentric and vice versa
7. Do not bounce, do not use momentum or rebound—but don't pause!
8. We arrive at the rep "turnaround" point and instantly switch directions
9. We save pausing for our intermediate template as an intensity amping tactic

PERIODIZED BEGINNER STRATEGY

Week 1	5 reps are done on all "top sets" on all exercises
Week 2	7-rep top set: we add two perfect reps to each top set
Week 3	9-rep top set: add two more perfect reps
Week 4	Begin anew: back to 5-rep sets, using a steeper angle
Week 5	7-rep top set: we add two perfect reps to each top set
Week 6	9-rep top set: add two more perfect reps
Week 7	Graduate to an intermediate CrossCore® regimen

BEGINNER TEMPLATE SUMMARY

EXERCISE SEQUENCE

SQUAT, TWO-LEG

CHEST PRESS, TWO-ARM

ROW, TWO-ARM

I-Y-T-RY

CURL, TWO-ARM

TRICEPS EXTENSION, TWO-ARM

DYNAMIC PLANK (KNEE-TUCK)

WEEK	REPS SET #1	REPS SET #2
1	5	5
2	5	7
3	5	9
4*	5	5
5	5	7
6	5	9

*Week 4 starts over using a steeper angle (more resistance)

INTERMEDIATE:
CROSSCORE® TRAINING SPLIT

How best do we construct an intermediate training template? We have peaked on our beginner routine, we have wrung all the gains possible out of it and the template no longer suffices; we need to jolt the body out of its rut. We seek two things: we want workout contrast and we need to increase the training *intensity*. We seek ways to make things different and variety provides the contrast we seek. One surefire way to institute contrast is to alter the exercises.

Philosophically and structurally, the beginner template is the ideal way to learn the core CrossCore® progressive resistance techniques. What better immersion, what better way to learn and ingrain the ultra-basic CrossCore® exercises than to do them two or three times a week, for weeks on end? After four to six weeks of performing the same core, ultra-basic CrossCore® exercises a trainee comes to a deep understanding of those movements. Perfect technique in the core CrossCore® exercises is imprinted. Time for phase II.

What better way to create contrast then to add new exercises? Let us learn radical new technical variations of the core CrossCore® exercise already learned. As an intermediate CrossCore® HardCore trainee, we are suddenly exposed to the idea of working one limb at a time, one arm or one leg, instability is bought to the forefront as we take the inherent instability of the CrossCore® and create more instability. We purposefully push and pull with all our might, but now on one leg, or with one arm. What better way to create contrast then to add new exercises? Let us learn radical new technical variations of the core CrossCore® exercise already learned. As an intermediate CrossCore® HardCore trainee, we are suddenly exposed to the idea of working one limb at a time, one arm or one leg, instability is bought to the forefront as we take the inherent instability of the CrossCore® and create more instability. We purposefully push and pull with all our might, but now on one leg, or with one arm.

THE WORKOUT

Monday
Airborne Squat (each leg), I-Y-T-rY, Seated Dips, Curl,
Single arm (each arm), Knee raise

Wednesday
Chest press, single arm (each arm), Row, one arm (each arm),
Front raise (I- part), Leg curl, Dynamic Plank (pike)

Friday
Pistol Squat (each leg), Extended Chest Press, I-Y-T-rY, single arm (each arm),
Curl, two arm, Triceps Press

WORKOUT FACTOIDS

To create the variety and intensity needed, we devise an intermediate workout template that differs dramatically from the beginner template. The needed contrast comes from the introduction of new exercises and new ways of doing old exercises. The intermediate may select one of the following workout strategies...

Straight set strategy: Attack each exercise separately; first set, easy reps using a gentle angle, a full ROM and grind rep speed; on the second set, optimally, we barely complete the final assigned rep of the 'all out set.' We perform two sets of each exercise, then move on; allow breathing to normalize between sets and one to two minutes between exercises.

Drop-set strategy: Perform *three* rapid-fire sets for each exercise; select a moderate to tough angle and rep to failure, move your feet to make payload lighter, rep out again; move feet to make payload *lighter* and rep to failure a third and final time. Finish one exercise drop set style, before moving onto the next. This is a three-phase drop set.

Giant set strategy: String exercises together and execute exercises in succession: in Monday's workout, airborne squats, lying leg curls, I-Y-T-r-Y, seated dips, curls and knee raise are all performed, one after another, without pause. Exercises done one after the other constitutes one "giant set." Perform two giant sets with two to five minutes' rest between sets: one light exercise cycle, rest, then one final, all-out exercise cycle/set.

Rotate and experiment with these three cornerstone progressive-resistance attack strategies, as applied to our new resistance tool: the CrossCore®.

INTERMEDIATE CROSSCORE® TRAINING STRATEGY

We inject variety into the intermediate CrossCore® training template by incorporating different exercises: stable two-handed and two-legged exercises are suddenly "switched out" for one-handed versions and variants; brand new movements are added. Each exercise session is different; no longer are we doing the same things three times a week. While the exercises might be different, we still must generate tremendous physical effort, we need struggle to complete reps, if we are to trigger muscle growth. We have one tremendous intensity booster that we have been 'saving.' We now utilize this tactic to amp-up the training intensity. We will now pause every time a rep switches from eccentric to concentric: we now pause at the 'turn-around.'

Pauses: intensity enhancer without peer. There is a strong case to be made that when using the CrossCore® as a resistance-training tool, pauses, along with grind rep speed and full range-of-motion, should be taught from day one. On the other hand, there is an equally persuasive school of thought that holds, why not "hold" pause reps in reserve for the intermediate phase? That still leaves the beginner to contend with perfecting techniques, the grind rep speed and a full ROM. Then, upon "graduating" from the beginner phase (after four to six weeks) add those "saved" pauses—in doing so, we ensure we achieve the next upward level of intensity needed to trigger growth and adaptation.

On all the exercises we add a pause when eccentric becomes concentric. How long should a pause be? Hardly long at all. Dorian Yates called his pauses, "Barely paused." We pause just long enough to halt any momentum. Too long a pause reduces poundage and rep capacity by an unacceptable degree. Proper pausing makes any exercise 20-50% more difficult—and that is sufficient. Slow the rep speed too much and the amount of poundage a person can handle is so dramatically reduced that all the bone-building, tendon and ligament thickening and strengthening is completely lost.

PERIODIZED INTERMEDIATE STRATEGY

Pause everything! In addition to using a full range-of-motion and grind rep speed, we now add pauses on all reps on all exercises. We use the identical week-by-week periodized "rep" strategy. Since the exercises are different, the rep strategy of adding two reps per week in 'wave' fashion, will work yet again. While the exercises are new, fresh and different, the set and rep template allows a feeling of familiarity. We know this strategy and now we apply it to a new batch of fresh and exciting exercises.

Week 1	5 reps are done on all "top sets" on all exercises
Week 2	7-rep top set: we add two perfect reps to each top set
Week 3	9-rep top set: add two more perfect reps
Week 4	Begin anew: back to 5-rep sets, use a steeper angle
Week 5	7-rep top set: we add two perfect reps to each top set
Week 6	9-rep top set: add two more perfect reps
Week 7	Graduate to an advanced CrossCore® regimen

INTERMEDIATE TEMPLATE SUMMARY

EXERCISE SEQUENCE

MONDAY	WEDNESDAY	FRIDAY
AIRBORNE SQUAT (EACH LEG)	CHEST PRESS, SINGLE ARM (EACH ARM)	PISTOL SQUAT (EACH LEG)

I-Y-T-RY	ROW, ONE ARM (EACH ARM)	EXTENDED CHEST PRESS

SEATED DIPS	FRONT RAISE (I- PART)	I-Y-T-RY, SINGLE ARM (EACH ARM)

CURL, SINGLE ARM (EACH ARM)	LEG CURL	CURL, TWO ARM

KNEE RAISE	DYNAMIC PLANK (PIKE)	TRICEPS PRESS

WEEK	REPS SET #1	REPS SET #2
1	5	5
2	5	7
3	5	9
4*	5	5
5	5	7
6	5	9

Same rotation of weeks
and reps as in beginners phase

*Week 4 starts over using a steeper
angle (more resistance)

ADVANCED:
CROSSCORE® TRAINING SPLIT

After months of training, after having 'mined' all the potential progress out of beginner and intermediate training templates, how then do we 'up the ante' to create advanced CrossCore® training templates? What can we do to make the hard harder and difficult even more so? How can the intermediate CrossCore® user take progress to the next level and trigger further muscle, power and strength gains?

New exercises and new levels of intensity are required yet again. More dramatic and radical strategies are invoked. Once again, at some point the intermediate training template ceases delivering tangible results, no matter how hard or how diligently the intermediate trains, at some point the body neutralizes the 'training effect' of the second stage routine. No problem, pros recognize stagnation (real pros anticipate stagnation before it occurs) and rotate in another equally effective training routine, but one that dramatically contrasts the routine it is replacing.

So how do we amp up the intensity? What new exercises and strategies do we have for the advanced CrossCore® trainee? Training routines are not created in a vacuum: we seek to construct a routine that is effective in that it covers all the muscular and physiological bases. In addition, regardless the exercises selected, we understand the need to generate effort, to purposefully struggle with the final reps of a set as this is where the progress resides. Here is one possible training routine in a universe of routine possibilities.

THE WORKOUT

Monday
Compound Squat (each leg), Rotational Chest Press, Curl, single arm (each arm)
Triceps Press (Single Arm), Dynamic plank (oblique)

Tuesday
I-Y-T-rY, single arm (each arm), Rotational Extended Row (each arm),
Leg curl, Leg Raises

Thursday
Pistol Squat (weight vest), Chest Press (weight vest), Curl, single arm (each arm)

Friday
Row, two arm (weight vest), I-Y-T-rY (steep angle),
Suspended Dip, Dynamic Plank (pike)

Wednesday, Saturday and Sunday: OFF

WORKOUT FACTOIDS

The idea with this particular advanced template was to engage in four, short, super intense CrossCore® sessions for a four to six week period. Each of the four training sessions lasts less than 15 minutes and the weekly cumulative training 'time under tension' (time spent actually using the CrossCore®) is less than 60 minutes—next to nothing when compared to the results derived. While this template does not require a lot of time, for it to be successful, it needs to be extremely *intense*. We can get away with short infrequent sessions but the tradeoff is ball-busting physical effort.

In each of these advanced movements, the rep ideal is to *barely* be able to complete the pre-assigned final rep on the top set: if the rep target is five, then ideally we barely complete the fifth rep—there is no sense even attempting rep six because the athlete has just completely exhausted his quotient of strength and he knows it. The targeted muscles are traumatized, literally, by the intensity of the effort. This degree of effort is required to trigger the muscle adaptation and growth we seek from our resistance training efforts.

ADVANCED TRAINING STRATEGY

The advanced CrossCore® user has much more latitude when compared to the rank beginner. By the time the CrossCore® user progresses to the advanced level, they will have a lot of sets and reps, a lot of exercises and angles under their belt. They will know their way around the tool and will have long-since mastered the core techniques and their sophisticated variants. Sets and reps, strength strategies (straight sets, giant sets, drop sets, etc.,) can be alternated workout to workout—as long as the CrossCore® user understands the goal of triggering hypertrophy, the *contents* of the workout can be shifted and changed at will.

1.   This particular *training split* calls for three weekly sessions
2.   Advanced techniques are used in every instance
3.   The targeted muscles are taken to capacity (and past) on all-out top sets
4.   We do not have to miss a rep to know not to undertake it

ADVANCED PERIODIZED TEMPLATE

These programming examples only scratch the surface of the possibilities with this versatile device. The periodized pre-planning variables are endless: tweak techniques, frequency, sets, reps, rep speed, number of cycles... Customize your training regimen to fit the peculiarities and particulars of your lifestyle. Properly sculpt the programming and reach your predefined goal. We need to be motivated, systematic, and understand how to use the CrossCore® to our best advantage.

*Allow us to introduce you to the idea of wearing a 'weighted backpack.' Just as the phrase suggests, we wrap a 10, 25, 35 or 45-pound barbell plate inside a blanket, stuff the blanket-wrapped plate into a backpack, put the backpack on and commence the CrossCore® exercise. Only now you push, pull or rotate with payload 10-45 pounds heavier than before, making things much, much harder. Alternately, the athlete could wear a weighted vest—though we have found the awkward nature of the backpack (all the weight is attached to the upper back) makes backpack payloads feel much heavier than the evenly distributed weighted vest. Any well-made backpack will do—the weighted back pack opens up an entire universe of payload-amping possibilities.

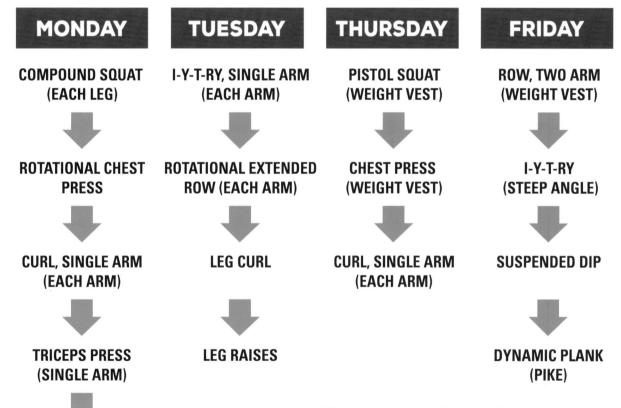

ADVANCED TEMPLATE SUMMARY

EXERCISE SEQUENCE

MONDAY	TUESDAY	THURSDAY	FRIDAY
COMPOUND SQUAT (EACH LEG)	I-Y-T-RY, SINGLE ARM (EACH ARM)	PISTOL SQUAT (WEIGHT VEST)	ROW, TWO ARM (WEIGHT VEST)
⬇	⬇	⬇	⬇
ROTATIONAL CHEST PRESS	ROTATIONAL EXTENDED ROW (EACH ARM)	CHEST PRESS (WEIGHT VEST)	I-Y-T-RY (STEEP ANGLE)
⬇	⬇	⬇	⬇
CURL, SINGLE ARM (EACH ARM)	LEG CURL	CURL, SINGLE ARM (EACH ARM)	SUSPENDED DIP
⬇	⬇		⬇
TRICEPS PRESS (SINGLE ARM)	LEG RAISES		DYNAMIC PLANK (PIKE)
⬇			
DYNAMIC PLANK (OBLIQUE)			

The advanced template should use 2 sets per exercise and 5-9 reps per set depending on goals. Decide on the number of reps prior to exercising and adjust the intensity to *barely complete* the final rep of each set.

PROGRAMMING ATHLETIC VERSUS MILITARY ARCHETYPES

I train active duty spec ops warriors and make myself available to these modern day samurai on an ongoing weekly basis. All have been exposed to my Old School strength methods firsthand. I work with spec ops commandos from other countries and I also work with counter-terrorism government types. I have been working with elite military long enough to understand their needs and limitations. When it comes to constructing strength programs that work for them, the military archetype has specific requirements.

I work with elite athletes involved in various sports and disciplines on an ongoing and continual basis. Just as the military archetype has needs and limitations, so too does the athletic archetype. What both athlete and warrior want from me is always the same: power, muscle and strength. I am not a strength and conditioning coach; I am not a strength-endurance coach; I am not a bodybuilder and I am not "fitness" instructor. My pie-sliver of expertise is pure power...

1.   How do we dramatically enhance our current quotient of pure physical power?
2.   How do we maximize our raw strength and build lean muscle mass?

Strong is my specialty. We make the best in the world stronger and we make them more muscular and we make them far more powerful; then we send them on their way back to do what they do, only now they will do it better.

I have devised a minimalistic, honed and pared, radically streamlined strength training system that was a perfect fit for time-pressed spec ops types. These men understand the need for pure power—but have limited time to train. The question they asked me was, how little weight training can a man do and still optimize his strength? It is not that they don't like strength training (they love it) it is that they are required to master and participate in so many other drills and escapades that time is the most precious and valued commodity.

We created a military template adopted for the spec ops archetype: they needed a time-compressed approach that could be customized according to current job demands; flexible, expandable, contractible, our approach could be done if the athlete could only train once a week or, if bored and with time on their hands, could be expanded. Frequency was an issue for these men. Some weeks they had all the time in the world, other weeks they had none. I created an 'elastic template.' Without going into workout content, which they would tweak according to goal and time, the flexibility in frequency was a big hit...in a nutshell...

If you have....	Length of strength training session
One day per week to train	one 45-minute session
Two days per week to train	two 30-minute sessions
Three days per week to train	three 20-minute sessions
Four days per week to train	four 15-minutes sessions
Five days per week to train	five 12-minute sessions
Six days per week to train	six 10-minute sessions

As a Korean intelligence officer told me after he used this approach, "You have many ways to smoke the cat out of the bag." We increase their raw power and usable, athletically applicable strength, yet we do so in a relatively short amount of time, typically eight to 16 weeks with 12 weeks being the average. We establish realistic short-term goals and we establish realistic long-term goals, based on the warrior/athlete's current strength levels, degree of expertise and realistic goals. We establish initial performance benchmarks in a wide range of movements and categories and then set our predetermined goals into a specific timeframe. We create achievable weekly mini-goals.

Recently we worked with an athlete that had been bench pressing 205 for five strict reps. By altering his technique, by increasing his training poundage a scant five pounds per week, he was able to stair-step his strength upward each week for 12 consecutive weeks. He ended by bench pressing 255 for five reps; not coincidentally, he added eight pounds of muscle and lost six pounds of body fat in the same timeframe. His bench press strength increased by an astounding 25% and his results are not atypical.

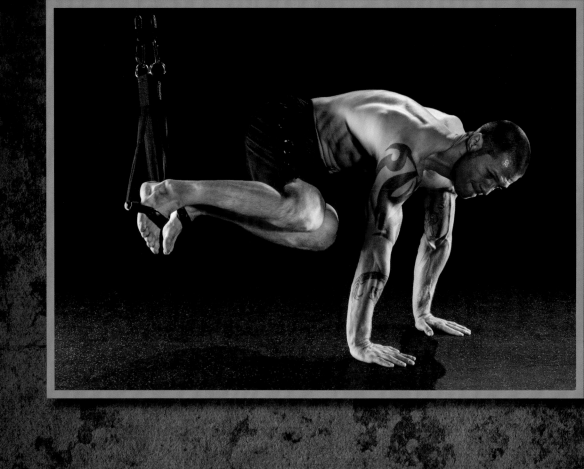

CONCLUSION

"TELL THEM,
TELL THEM WHAT YOU
HAVE TOLD THEM—

—Aristotelian Triptych

n the end, after all the books have been read, after all the theories discussed, after all the debates debated, after all the workouts have been designed and after all the talk is talked, there is the training.

The best single piece of progressive resistance training advice I can ever give you is to train hard. How *hard* is "hard enough?" We seek a degree of training effort that is nothing less than Herculean. Our physical efforts, our struggles, need be sufficiently intense in order to attain hormonal critical mass: when our efforts are truly Herculean, the body releases protective endorphins. How do you know what that occurs?

You feel it. You get a perceptible internal glow. No need to search, no need to ponder, the endorphin 'rush' either occurs or it doesn't, you either experience it or you don't. It is not a subtle thing: an endorphin rush is a tsunami, a hormonal acid trip.

Most normal humans never experience a single endorphin rush in their entire lives. They never have a need to. Modern life is insular, sissified, devoid of Herculean physical exertion. In this day and age, there is never a need to equal or exceed physical capacities—ever. We might be stressed out of our minds, we might be emotionally whipsawed, psychologically devastated by life, but rarely if ever does modern man need to exert to the max, physically.

200 years ago, modern man's ancestors were cutting down logs with axes by hand to sculpt log cabins; they walked and ran and hunted and exerted and sweated, they ate organic and dieted periodically due to food shortages. Nowadays you might die of a heart attack or be racked with stress-induced peptic ulcers, but you do not get thrown from a horse full gallop while chasing a bear with a musket. We do not wrangle cattle and fight Indians.

Modern man is ignorant of the endorphin/hypertrophy connection. Modern fitness experts, who should be alerting, pointing out this benchmark to their high-paying clients and followers, remain blissfully ignorant of this benchmark phenomenon. Regardless the resistance-training tool, it is the degree of pure physical effort that obtains the desired results we seek.

There is no missing or overlooking the endorphin "glow"—it is as real and tangible as hunger, as a sex urge or as anger or rage. If you are puzzled by this crazy hormone talk, then you have not experienced the post-workout endorphin glow we speak of. Elite athletes not only know of the effort-induced endorphin glow, they use its appearance (or non-appearance) as a workout benchmark. They seek to train hard enough in every session to trigger the release of endorphins. The absence is viewed with cause for alarm that the degree of effort was insufficient and therefore the entire training session wasted effort.

The elite understand that endorphins are the precursor to hypertrophy: without the presence of endorphins, there is no hypertrophy. Does this all this seem nebulous, fuzzy and indistinct? Only for those who have never experienced endorphin bliss.

In *resistance* training, the harder you train the greater the results. That which does not kill me makes me stronger—and more muscular.

Regardless the tool, severity of effort is inexorably linked to the successful attainment of all the wonderful physical attributes proper progressive resistance training bestows. The tool selected is secondary to the effort generated. You can fail to trigger hypertrophy using the most sophisticated of devices and you can trigger hypertrophy with the crudest of devices. Use the most perfect of techniques in sub-maximal fashion and acquire subpar results.

Use the crudest tool imaginable with savage intensity (and good technique) and reap a muscle and power windfall.

One cursory look at the muscled-up bodies created in prison verifies the prime commandment of power: in resistance training, intensity, degree of effort, trumps everything. Prisoners nationwide are uniformly making outstanding gains and their gains are rooted in two things: intensity or effort and consistency of effort. These men train hard as hell and never have to miss a training session.

Prisoners use the worst possible collection of training tools (or are they?) and endure the worst possible nutrition—prison chow gruel. Yet across the entire correctional system, in any prison that allows barbells and benches, chin and dip bars, prisoners are making gains and building muscular bodies that shame free men worldwide.

What's the takeaway? When you use the CrossCore®, seek ways to make your training exercises maximally intense, intense enough to trigger the always-detectable endorphin benchmark. Be consistent. Don't miss sessions.

A resistance tool need be combined with techniques designed to stimulate the maximum number of muscle fibers. We hone and refine specific techniques in order to elicit specific physiological results. We create and master these techniques and we never cease to seek to improve upon them.

Every technique has (or should have) a technical archetype: we seek to emulate these archetypes to ever-greater degrees of technical exactitude. Over time we refine and hone exercise techniques.

When it comes to resistance *training*, effective resistance training, muscle-building, strength-infusing resistance training, the CrossCore® can be an effective, result-producing tool—in the hands of an expert using our HardCore strategy.

This book shows you how to obtain outstanding resistance results from a new tool utilizing new techniques and old school tactics, expropriated from hardcore weight training and reapplied for use with the CrossCore®.

We live in Real World, the world of delivered gains, not promised gains; the folks we work with are national and world level. Regardless their respective specialty, they seek us out to help in making them *radically stronger.*

The only thing that matters to these people is results—does the tool and strategy obtain the results promised? Yes or no?

If the answer is yes, then that tool or system gets included in the arsenal of effective modes and methods an athlete keeps in their quiver of proven-effective strategies. As the elite know, there is no single mode or method that trumps all others; no single system renders all other systems obsolete and ineffectual. That is not the way it works.

The elite athlete knows better. The elite have a wide selection of proven-effective resistance routines, ones they have used successfully in the past. They periodically and systematically rotate strength systems, squeezing all the gains out of a particular system within a particular timeframe before placing the now-burnt out system back in the "strength closet," like a shirt back from the dry cleaners, for future effective use, somewhere down the road.

The human body loves hemostasis, sameness, normalcy, and seeks to neutralize any 'training effect.' When a new and intense resistance system is successfully instituted, the body immediately attempts to cope and adapt to this new and traumatic form of self-inflicted physical stress. The body seeks to adapt to this new type and degree of stress; the body seeks to neutralize the trauma. Yet in an unfunny iron irony, when the trauma is neutralized, muscle gains and strength gains cease. The elite recognize this physiological fact of life.

We need a closet full of training modes and methods, all proven, all well thought-out and battle-tested.

1. Select a realistic goal
2. Set that goal into a periodized time frame
3. Set up the training template
4. Pick the tool and
5. Create the workout content

Now it's time to train. Now is when the rubber meets the road. All the talked is talked, all the strategies decided on, all the thoughts thought: now it is time for you to jump into the deep end of the pool.

When you finally wrap your fists around the two handles of CrossCore®, once all the fooling around is over, once it is time to really *train*, then it is time to embrace the philosophic and psychological concept of *struggle*. And effort. And intensity.

Without struggle, without intense physical effort, without the mental toughness to absorb some discomfort, without consistency and tenacity—you will gain nothing from your resistance training efforts. You might as well go bowling or play a round of golf or go garden. Without intense physical effort, without struggle, then the CrossCore® ceases to have any resistance training benefit.

Most "fitness" devotees never progress past a certain level because they are ignorant of the need for intense effort—or incapable of generating the requisite degree of effort, the sheer struggle and intensity needed to make resistance training sessions effective and productive.

You no longer have the excuse of ignorance because you are reading these words.

Dating back to Grecian times—before microphones, acoustically tuned halls, and auditoriums were invented—the Rule of Three was often used by playwrights and actors in order that all sections of the audience would be able to follow along. The actor would say the line three times, expressed differently stage left, then straight ahead and finally stage right. Said differently with the same meaning three times.

Most Grecian plays were performed outdoors in amphitheater and expressing a plot device three times allowed the entire crowd to follow the action. Clever playwrights became adept at repetition. Handled deftly, imaginative repetition enhances and reinforces a storyline.

When using this fabulous tool in a very specific way to elicit very specific results we adhere to the rule of threes. This strange and wonderful device teleports the user into an exercise universe that is inaccessible by any other tool. The rotational universe available with the CrossCore® is absolutely unobtainable using any other tool.

No other tool, device or machine allows the trainee the ability to lighten and groove in a technique with the ease and sophistication of a properly-used CrossCore®.   No other device enables you to alter resistance mid-rep, and only the CrossCore® allows the user access to this unique and infinite universe of rotational exercise possibilities.

Used with HardCore protocols, the CrossCore® will deliver results...

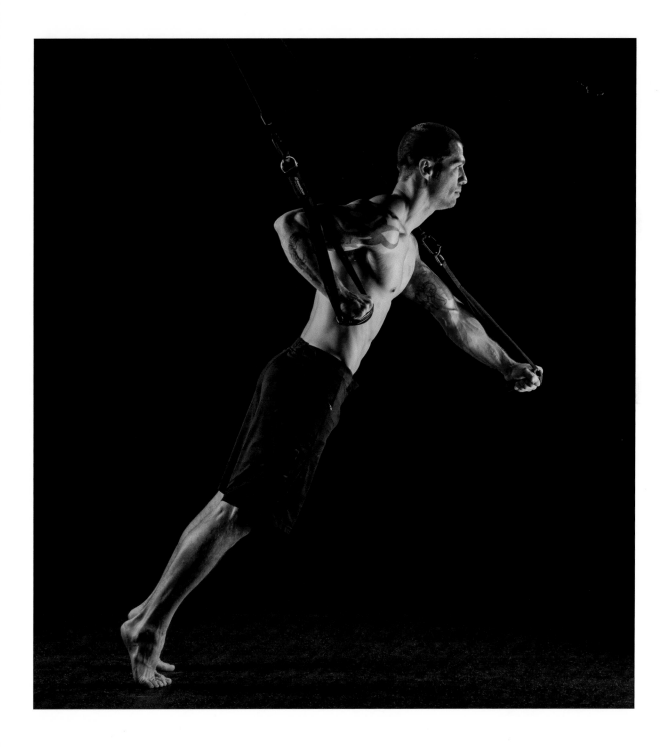

ABOUT THE AUTHORS

MARTY GALLAGHER

   Marty Gallagher has been involved in high-level athletics for over 50 years. He captured his first national title and set his first national records as a 17-year old teenage Olympic weightlifter in 1967. In May of 2013 he set his most recent national records as a 64-year old powerlifter. He won the 1992 IPF world masters powerlifting title and has taken silver and bronze medals in world championships. He is a six-time national champion masters powerlifter.

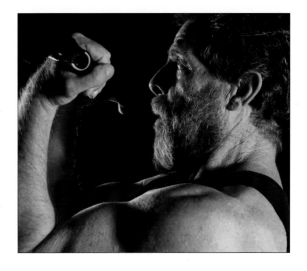

   As a coach he guided Team USA to the IPF world team title in 1991 and coached Black's gym to five national powerlifting team titles. He was mentored by the 1st world powerlifting champion Hugh "Huge" Cassidy and Gallagher in turn mentored hall-of-fame powerlifting world dominator "Captain" Kirk Karwoski. Gallagher competition coached Ed "King" Coan, the world's greatest powerlifter, along with iron immortals Doug Furnas, Lamar Gant and Mark Chaillet. Marty works with the military elite spec ops fighters (in this country and abroad) along with governmental special units within various agencies.

   As a writer Gallagher is widely read and considered one of the finest writers operating within the health, nutrition, bodybuilding, strength and athletic training genre. He has had over 1,000 articles published since 1978, including 232 weekly 'ask the expert' fitness columns for the *Washington Post. com* and 89 articles published during a ten year relationship with *Muscle & Fitness* and *Flex* magazine. Gallagher's biographic on Ed Coan was called, "the greatest powerlifting book ever written," by the late Joe Weider. Rock star Henry Rollins called the Coan book, "Awesome!" Dr. Jeff Everson described Gallagher's Magnus opus, **The Purposeful Primitive** "A literary masterpiece." Gallagher lives in rural Pennsylvania.

CHRISTOPHER G. HARDY, D.O., MPH, CSCS

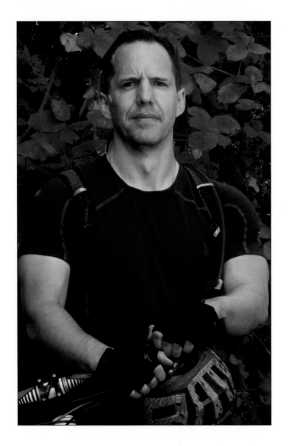

Dr. Chris Hardy is emerging as a leader in public health, merging his expertise in nutrition, strength and conditioning, and in clinical and preventive medicine into a comprehensive approach to treat chronic disease.

Dr. Hardy has a diverse background, including 13 years active military service in both the U.S. Army and U.S. Navy. He is a previous graduate of the Naval Diving and Salvage Training Center and Underwater Construction Basic Course, going on to serve as a military deep sea diver. He left the military the first time after four years of service to start his higher education.

Dr. Hardy is a graduate of Old Dominion University, earning a bachelor of science in biochemistry. He went on to medical school at WVSOM in Lewisburg WV, graduating as a Doctor of Osteopathic Medicine.

After medical school and internship, Dr. Hardy re-entered the military as a Navy physician, serving aboard the USS WASP (LHD-1) as medical officer and joining the ship on deployment in support of Operation Enduring Freedom. He then served another operational tour as a medical officer before attending Johns Hopkins University for medical specialty training.

Dr. Hardy completed his specialty training in Occupational and Environmental Medicine at the Johns Hopkins School of Public Health where he served as Chief Resident, also earning a Master of Public Health degree with a concentration in toxicology.

Dr. Hardy is Board Certified in Occupational and Environmental Medicine under the American College of Preventive Medicine. He has also completed formal training in medical acupuncture and is a Certified Strength and Conditioning Specialist by the NSCA. He is currently enrolled in the Fellowship in Integrative Medicine at the University of Arizona.

Chris lives in Everett Washington and is passionate about guitars, mountain biking, and health and wellness. He is still active as a trainer and gives nutrition lectures around the local community. He is married to his talented wife Carrie, a former biochemist and current student in Naturopathic Medicine at Bastyr University. His daughter Anna is a graduate student in Geophysics at Virginia Tech University.

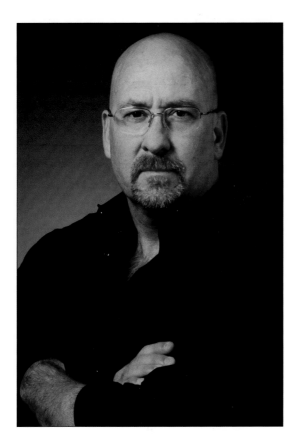

MICHAEL KRIVKA

Michael A. Krivka, Sr. is a Washington, DC native who has been training and teaching Russian Kettlebell since 2001 and a Master RKC. As one of the most highly reviewed kettlebell instructors in the world on the Dragon Door Web site, he is also a highly sought after instructor and has traveled coast-to-coast teaching kettlebells to a wide variety of people (SWAT/SERT teams, USMC officers, MMA and BJJ practitioners and even "Soccer Moms and Dads"). In addition, he is the author of a bestselling e-book *Code Name: Indestructible*, is a regular contributor to the Dragon Door website, and is featured in several upcoming instructional videos and books. He is also a lifelong martial artist with over 30 years of training in Jeet June Do / JKD Concepts and the Filipino Martial Arts (Kali, Escrima and Arnis) where he is a Full Instructor under Guro Dan Inosanto.

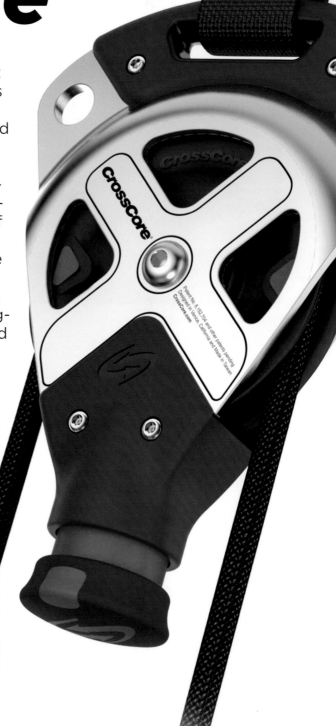
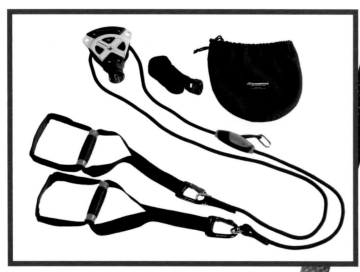

www.facebook.com/DragonDoorPublications

Keep Abreast of Dragon Door's Latest Articles, Interviews, Products, Workshops And Other Breaking News on Our Official Facebook Page.

Plus: Get Special Dragon Door Facebook-Only Offers.

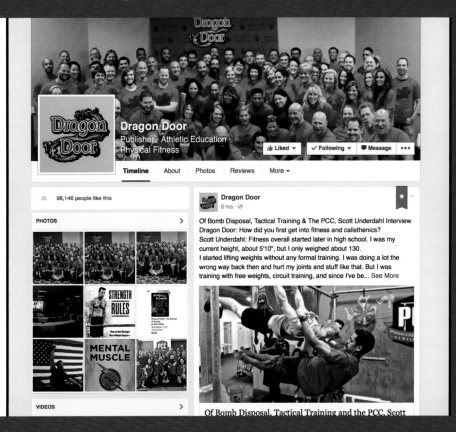

http://kbforum.dragondoor.com

Kettlebells? Strength? Bodyweight? Conditioning? Diet?—Get Your Questions Answered by the Experts on DragonDoor.com's Premier Forums

And Join Discussions, Stay Informed About Hot New Training Resources and Opportunities...

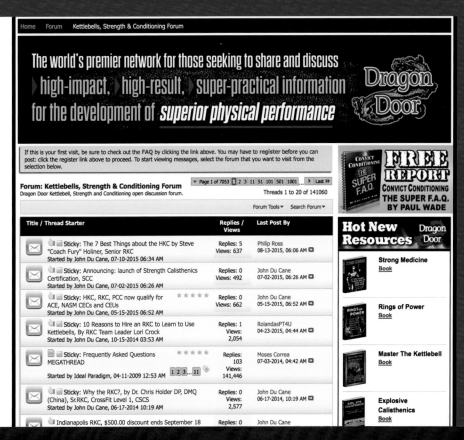

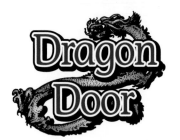

1·800·899·5111

24 HOURS A DAY • FAX YOUR ORDER (866) 280-7619

ORDERING INFORMATION

Telephone Orders For faster service you may place your orders by calling Toll Free 24 hours a day, 7 days a week, 365 days per year. When you call, please have your credit card ready.

Customer Service Questions? Please call us between 9:00am– 11:00pm EST Monday to Friday at 1-800-899-5111. Local and foreign customers call 513-346-4160 for orders and customer service

100% One-Year Risk-Free Guarantee. If you are not completely satisfied with any product—we'll be happy to give you a prompt exchange, credit, or refund, as you wish. Simply return your purchase to us, and please let us know why you were dissatisfied--it will help us to provide better products and services in the future. Shipping and handling fees are non-refundable.

Complete and mail with full payment to: Dragon Door Publications, 5 County Road B East, Suite 3, Little Canada, MN 55117

Please print clearly

Sold To: **A**

Name_____

Street_____

City_____

State _____ Zip _____

Day phone*_____

* Important for clarifying questions on orders

Please print clearly

Sold To: (Street address for delivery)   **B**

Name_____

Street_____

City_____

State _____ Zip _____

Email_____

Warning to foreign customers: The Customs in your country may or may not tax or otherwise charge you an additional fee for goods you receive. Dragon Door Publications is charging you only for U.S. handling and international shipping. Dragon Door Publications is in no way responsible for any additional fees levied by Customs, the carrier or any other entity.

Item #	Qty.	Item Description	Item Price	A or B	Total

HANDLING AND SHIPPING CHARGES • NO CODS

Total Amount of Order Add (Excludes kettlebells and kettlebell kits):

$00.00 to 29.99	**Add $7.00**	$100.00 to 129.99	**Add $14.00**
$30.00 to 49.99	**Add $6.00**	$130.00 to 169.99	**Add $16.00**
$50.00 to 69.99	**Add $8.00**	$170.00 to 199.99	**Add $18.00**
$70.00 to 99.99	**Add $11.00**	$200.00 to 299.99	**Add $20.00**
		$300.00 and up	**Add $24.00**

Canada and Mexico add $6.00 to US charges. All other countries, flat rate, double US Charges. See Kettlebell section for Kettlebell Shipping and handling charges.

Total of Goods	
Shipping Charges	
Rush Charges	
Kettlebell Shipping Charges	
OH residents add 6.5% sales tax	
MN residents add 6.5% sales	

METHOD OF PAYMENT ___Check ___M.O. ___Mastercard ___Visa ___Discover ___Amex

Account No. (Please indicate all the numbers on your credit card)   EXPIRATION DATE

▢▢▢▢ ▢▢▢▢ ▢▢▢▢ ▢▢▢▢   ▢▢/▢▢

Day Phone: _____

Signature: _____ Date: _____

NOTE: We ship best method available for your delivery address. Foreign orders are sent by air. Credit card or International M.O. only. **For RUSH processing** of your order, add an additional $10.00 per address. Available on money order & charge card orders only.

Errors and omissions excepted. Prices subject to change without notice.

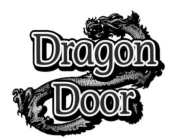

1·800·899·5111

24 HOURS A DAY • FAX YOUR ORDER (866) 280-7619

O R D E R I N G   I N F O R M A T I O N

Telephone Orders For faster service you may place your orders by calling Toll Free 24 hours a day, 7 days a week, 365 days per year. When you call, please have your credit card ready.

Customer Service Questions? Please call us between 9:00am– 11:00pm EST Monday to Friday at 1-800-899-5111. Local and foreign customers call 513-346-4160 for orders and customer service

100% One-Year Risk-Free Guarantee. If you are not completely satisfied with any product—we'll be happy to give you a prompt exchange, credit, or refund, as you wish. Simply return your purchase to us, and please let us know why you were dissatisfied--it will help us to provide better products and services in the future. Shipping and handling fees are non-refundable.

Complete and mail with full payment to: Dragon Door Publications, 5 County Road B East, Suite 3, Little Canada, MN 55117

Please print clearly
Sold To: A

Name_____

Street_____

City_____

State_____ Zip_____

Day phone*_____

* Important for clarifying questions on orders

Please print clearly
Sold To: (Street address for delivery)   B

Name_____

Street_____

City_____

State_____ Zip_____

Email_____

Warning to foreign customers: The Customs in your country may or may not tax or otherwise charge you an additional fee for goods you receive. Dragon Door Publications is charging you only for U.S. handling and international shipping. Dragon Door Publications is in no way responsible for any additional fees levied by Customs, the carrier or any other entity.

ITEM #	QTY.	ITEM DESCRIPTION	ITEM PRICE	A OR B	TOTAL

HANDLING AND SHIPPING CHARGES • NO CODS

Total Amount of Order Add (Excludes kettlebells and kettlebell kits):

$00.00 to 29.99	**Add $7.00**	**$100.00 to 129.99**	**Add $14.00**
$30.00 to 49.99	**Add $6.00**	**$130.00 to 169.99**	**Add $16.00**
$50.00 to 69.99	**Add $8.00**	**$170.00 to 199.99**	**Add $18.00**
$70.00 to 99.99	**Add $11.00**	**$200.00 to 299.99**	**Add $20.00**
		$300.00 and up	**Add $24.00**

Canada and Mexico add $6.00 to US charges. All other countries, flat rate, double US Charges. See Kettlebell section for Kettlebell Shipping and handling charges.

Total of Goods	
Shipping Charges	
Rush Charges	
Kettlebell Shipping Charges	
OH residents add 6.5% sales	
tax	
MN residents add 6.5% sales	

METHOD OF PAYMENT ___Check ___M.O. ___Mastercard ___Visa ___Discover ___Amex

Account No. (Please indicate all the numbers on your credit card)   EXPIRATION DATE

☐☐☐☐ ☐☐☐☐ ☐☐☐☐ ☐☐☐☐   ☐☐/☐☐

Day Phone: _____

Signature: _____ Date: _____

NOTE: We ship best method available for your delivery address. Foreign orders are sent by air. Credit card or International M.O. only. **For RUSH processing** of your order, add an additional $10.00 per address. Available on money order & charge card orders only.

Errors and omissions excepted. Prices subject to change without notice.